Compulsive Sexual Behavior Disorder

UNDERSTANDING, ASSESSMENT, AND TREATMENT

Compulsive Sexual Behavior Disorder

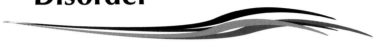

UNDERSTANDING, ASSESSMENT, AND TREATMENT

Edited by

Richard Balon, M.D.

Peer Briken, M.D.

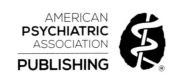

AMERICAN
PSYCHIATRIC
ASSOCIATION
PUBLISHING

25   24   23   22   21   5   4   3   2   1

American Psychiatric Association Publishing
800 Maine Avenue SW, Suite 900
Washington, DC 20024-2812
www.appi.org

Library of Congress Cataloging-in-Publication Data
Names: Balon, Richard, editor. | Briken, Peer, 1969- editor. | American Psychi-
    atric Association Publishing, issuing body.
Title: Compulsive sexual behavior disorder : understanding, assessment, and
    treatment / edited by Richard Balon, Peer Briken.
Description: First edition. | Washington, DC : American Psychiatric Association
    Publishing, [2021] | Includes bibliographical references and index.
Identifiers: LCCN 2020051930 (print) | LCCN 2020051931 (ebook) | ISBN
    9781615372195 (paperback ; alk. paper) | ISBN 9781615373789 (ebook)
Subjects: MESH: Sexual and Gender Disorders—psychology | Sexual and Gen-
    der Disorders—diagnosis | Sexual and Gender Disorders—therapy | Com-
    pulsive Behavior—psychology | Compulsive Behavior—diagnosis |
    Compulsive Behavior—therapy
Classification: LCC RC556 (print) | LCC RC556 (ebook) | NLM WM 611 |
    DDC 616.85/83—dc23
LC record available at https://lccn.loc.gov/2020051930
LC ebook record available at https://lccn.loc.gov/2020051931

British Library Cataloguing in Publication Data
A CIP record is available from the British Library.

Contents

Contributors

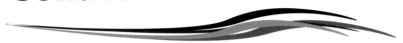

Bianca P. Acevedo, Ph.D.
Research Associate, Department of Psychological and Brain Sciences, University of California–Santa Barbara, Santa Barbara, California

Rafael Ballester-Arnal, Ph.D.
Full Professor, Department of Basic and Clinical Psychology and Psychobiology, Universitat Jaume I, Castellón de la Plana, Spain

Richard Balon, M.D.
Departments of Psychiatry and Behavioral Neurosciences and Anesthesiology, Wayne State University School of Medicine, Detroit, Michigan

Dianne Berg, Ph.D.
Assistant Professor, Program in Human Sexuality, Department of Family Medicine and Community Health, University of Minnesota, Minneapolis, Minnesota

Brad D. Booth, M.D., FRCPC
Forensic Psychiatrist, Integrated Forensic Program, Royal Ottawa Mental Health Centre; Associate Professor, Division of Forensic Psychiatry, Department of Psychiatry, University of Ottawa, Ontario, Canada

Peer Briken, M.D.
Institute for Sex Research, Sexual Medicine and Forensic Psychiatry, University Medical Center, Hamburg-Eppendorf, Germany

Leonardo Candelario-Perez, Ph.D.
Sexual Health Consultant, Health Partners, St Paul; Program in Human Sexuality, Department of Family Medicine and Community Health, University of Minnesota, Minneapolis, Minnesota

Patrick J. Carnes, Ph.D.
Founder, International Institute for Trauma and Addiction Professionals and Gentle Path Press, Carefree, Arizona

Eli Coleman, Ph.D.
Professor, Program in Human Sexuality, Department of Family Medicine and Community Health, University of Minnesota, Minneapolis, Minnesota

Kristian Daneback, Ph.D.
Full Professor, Department of Social Work, University of Gothenburg, Gothenburg, Sweden

Janna Dickenson, Ph.D.
Assistant Teaching Professor, Department of Psychology, University of California–San Diego, La Jolla, California; Program in Human Sexuality, Department of Family Medicine and Community Health, University of Minnesota, Minneapolis, Minnesota

Cristina Giménez-García, Ph.D.
Associate Professor, Department of Basic and Clinical Psychology and Psychobiology, Universitat Jaume I, Castelló de la Plana, Spain

Abby Girard, Psy.D.
Assistant Professor, Program in Human Sexuality, Department of Family Medicine and Community Health, University of Minnesota, Minneapolis, Minnesota

Mateusz Gola, Ph.D.
Associate Researcher, Institute for Neural Computations, University of California–San Diego, La Jolla, California; Associate Research Professor, Institute of Psychology, Polish Academy of Sciences, Warsaw, Poland

Meg S. Kaplan, Ph.D.

Clinical Professor of Psychology in Psychiatry, Department of Psychiatry, College of Physicians and Surgeons, Columbia University, New York, New York

Drew A. Kingston, C.Psych., Ph.D.

Adjunct Scientist, Integrated Forensic Program, Royal Ottawa Mental Health Centre, Ottawa, Ontario, Canada; Senior Clinical Director, HOPE program, San Diego, California

Verena Klein, Ph.D.

Postdoctoral Researcher, Institute for Sex Research and Forensic Psychiatry, University Medical Center, Hamburg, Germany

Alex Kovic, Psy.D.

Psychologist, Natalis Counseling and Psychology Solutions; Program in Human Sexuality, Department of Family Medicine and Community Health, University of Minnesota, Minneapolis, Minnesota

Shane W. Kraus, Ph.D.

Assistant Professor, Department of Psychology, University of Nevada–Las Vegas, Las Vegas, Nevada

Richard B. Krueger, M.D.

Department of Psychiatry, College of Physicians and Surgeons, Columbia University; Department of Psychiatry, New York-Presbyterian Hospital, New York State Psychiatric Institute, New York, New York

Mário Ferreira Lourenço, M.D., Ph.D.

Former Professor of Medical Psychology at Dentistry Faculty, Oporto University, Porto; Head, Couple Clinic, Hospital da Senhora da Oliveira, Guimarães; Former President, Portuguese Society of Clinical Sexology, Lisbon; Member, International Academy of Medical Sexology, Porto, Portugal

Rosemary Munns, Psy.D.

Assistant Professor, Program in Human Sexuality, Department of Family Medicine and Community Health, University of Minnesota, Minneapolis, Minnesota

António Pacheco Palha, M.D., Ph.D.

Full Professor of Psychiatry, Retired, FMUP; Former President, Portuguese Society of Psychiatry and Mental Health, Lisbon; Clinical Director, Casa de Saúde Bom Jesus (Hospitaller Sisters), Braga; President, Portuguese Language Mental Health Association, Porto, Portugal; Honorary Member, World Psychiatry Association, Geneva, Switzerland

Ami Popat-Jain, Ph.D.

Adjunct Professor, Department of Applied Psychology, Northeastern University, Boston, Massachusetts

Marc N. Potenza, M.D., Ph.D.

Professor of Psychiatry, Departments of Psychiatry and Neuroscience and Child Study Center, Yale University School of Medicine, New Haven; Director, Connecticut Mental Health Center, New Haven; Director, Connecticut Council on Problem Gambling, Wethersfield, Connecticut

G. Nic Rider, Ph.D.

Assistant Professor, Program in Human Sexuality, Department of Family Medicine and Community Health, University of Minnesota, Minneapolis, Minnesota

Kenneth Paul Rosenberg, M.D.

Clinical Associate Professor, Psychiatry, Weill Cornell University Medical Center and New York Presbyterian Hospital, New York

Daniel Turner, M.D., Ph.D.

Department of Psychiatry and Psychotherapy, University Medical Center, Mainz, Germany

Joel Watts, M.D., FRCPC

Clinical Director and Forensic Psychiatrist, Integrated Forensic Program, Royal Ottawa Mental Health Centre; Assistant Professor, Division of Forensic Psychiatry, Department of Psychiatry, University of Ottawa, Ontario, Canada

Foreword

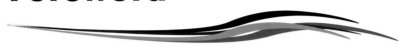

The diagnostic category of compulsive sexual behavior disorder (CSBD) has been included in the ICD-11 and thus is relatively new (Kraus et al. 2018). This construct replaces the older concept of excessive sexual drive, which was located in the chapter on sexual dysfunctions in the ICD-10 as the counterpart to hypoactive sexual desire disorder. The World Health Organization (WHO) has therefore taken a different approach from the American Psychiatric Association with regard to hypersexual disorder, which was not included in DSM-5 (American Psychiatric Association 2013; Kafka 2014). WHO included CSBD in its classification, listing it among impulse-control disorders.

For clinicians, patients with CSBD are a well-known group that has been described in the clinical literature for more than 100 years (Briken 2020). There has always been an accompanying risk that sexual behavior will be prematurely pathologized, and this applies to the current diagnosis of CSBD as well. However, this risk tends to decrease when an accurate description is available, which makes valid and reliable diagnosis much more likely than is possible with categories that are not described in detail, as was the case with the ICD-10 diagnosis. We believe that measurable progress has been made. In a Web-based field study comparing the diagnostic accuracy and clinical utility of some diagnoses using vignettes presented to health professionals from all WHO regions, the diagnostic accuracy of the ICD-11 was significantly higher for CSBD (89.3% correct diagnoses) than for the ICD-10's excessive sexual drive diagnosis (48.7%; $\chi^2[1] = 16.3$; $P < 0.001$) (Gaebel et al. 2020).

This book is therefore being published at just the right time, and it aims to offer clinicians of various specialties and disciplines (e.g., psychiatrists, sexual medicine specialists, gynecologists, family practitioners, psychologists) a practical introduction to the topic and its various facets. Our guiding question was: What does the clinician need to know in order to examine, assess, and treat patients with CSBD? We believed that the book should be practical, scientifically sound, and not too extensive. We hope that we succeeded.

We can distinguish CSBD, on the one hand, as an autoerotic activity form of sexual behavior and, on the other hand, as a sexual behavior that includes other people. For the former, the current consumption of pornography through digital media plays a special role. For the latter, partner-related sexual activities, such as promiscuous behavior, have been discussed in the past in connection with sexual risk behavior and the danger of sexually transmitted diseases. Many studies have been done about men who have sex with men (MSM) in this context. We do not include separate chapters on MSM or people with nonheterosexual orientations, but we do cover sexual minorities in the different chapters when it makes sense to do so. There are also no separate chapters and no differentiated mentioning of trans, intersex, and asexuality, because no studies have yet investigated these or other spectrums of sex or gender (Nieder et al. 2020) more specifically. We believe that issues of gender and sexual orientation are not salient for establishing the diagnosis of CSBD.

We hope that readers of this book will be those who come into contact with patients with CSBD in counseling, psychotherapy, sex therapy, or psychiatry. The book can be the basis for therapeutic and drug treatment and can provide good support for theoretical and practical training. We welcome feedback, suggestions for improvement, or practical advice from interested readers. We hope not only that the research activities in this field will continue to increase but also that patients will be able to find appropriate professional care. If the book can contribute to this goal, we will be satisfied. Above all, the book should serve patients with CSBD, who should not be restricted with moralizing, negative attitudes about their sexual behaviors but should be supported in finding a form of sexual health that satisfies them and frees them from distress.

Richard Balon, M.D., Detroit, Michigan
Peer Briken, M.D., Hamburg, Germany

REFERENCES

American Psychiatric Association: Diagnostic and Statistical Manual of Mental Disorders, 5th Edition. Washington, DC, American Psychiatric Association, 2013
Briken P: An integrated model to assess and treat compulsive sexual behaviour disorder. Nat Rev Urol 17(7):391–406, 2020

Gaebel W, Stricker J, Riesbeck M, et al: Accuracy of diagnostic classification and clinical utility assessment of ICD-11 compared to ICD-10 in 10 mental disorders: findings from a web-based field study. Eur Arch Psychiatry Clin Neurosci 270(3):281–289, 2020

Kafka MP: What happened to hypersexual disorder? Arch Sex Behav 43(7):1259–1261, 2014

Kraus SW, Krueger RB, Briken P, et al: Compulsive sexual behaviour disorder in the ICD-11. World Psychiatry 17(1):109–110, 2018

Nieder TO, Güldenring A, Woellert K, et al: Ethical aspects of mental health care for lesbian, gay, bi-, pan-, asexual, and transgender people: a case-based approach. Yale J Biol Med 93(4):593–602, 2020

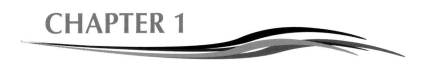

CHAPTER 1

Compulsive Sexual Behavior Disorder

FROM MYTHS TO REALITY

Richard Balon, M.D.
Peer Briken, M.D.

> More is lost by indecision than wrong decision. Indecision is the thief of opportunity. It will steal you blind.
>
> Marcus Tullius Cicero

The World Health Organization (WHO) released the 11th revision of its *International Classification of Diseases* (ICD-11) on June 18, 2018, and adopted it on May 25, 2019. ICD-11 will come into effect on January 1,

2022. One of the new diagnoses in ICD-11 is compulsive sexual behavior disorder (CSBD; 6C72), which is included among the impulse-control disorders. According to ICD-11 (World Health Organization 2019),

> Compulsive sexual behaviour disorder is characterised by a persistent pattern of failure to control intense, repetitive sexual impulses or urges resulting in repetitive sexual behaviour. Symptoms may include repetitive sexual activities becoming a central focus of the person's life to the point of neglecting health and personal care or other interests, activities and responsibilities; numerous unsuccessful efforts to significantly reduce repetitive sexual behaviour; and continued repetitive sexual behaviour despite adverse consequences or deriving little or no satisfaction from it. The pattern of failure to control intense, sexual impulses or urges and resulting repetitive sexual behaviour is manifested over an extended period of time (e.g., 6 months or more), and causes marked distress or significant impairment in personal, family, social, educational, occupational, or other important areas of functioning. Distress that is entirely related to moral judgments and disapproval about sexual impulses, urges, or behaviours is not sufficient to meet this requirement.

Paraphilias or paraphilic disorders are an exclusionary criterion of the CSBD diagnosis.

The CSBD diagnosis was and still is the subject of intensive debate. In his seminal review, Kafka (2010) summarized the existing literature on hypersexual behavior/diagnosis and proposed hypersexual disorder (HD) diagnostic criteria for DSM-5 (American Psychiatric Association 2013), with similarities to what we now call CSBD. He argued that HD should be included in DSM-5 and be classified as a sexual disorder. He wrote,

> Hypersexual Disorder has been primarily characterized as compulsive, impulsive, a behavioral addiction or a sexual desire disorder. Regarding the possible categorical placement in DSM-5, this author suggests that the term "compulsive," while apt in describing features of these conditions, is not consistent with prior DSM-based conceptualization of an obsessive-compulsive spectrum disorder. The categorization of Hypersexual Disorder as an impulsive-compulsive disorder or behavioral addiction in DSM-5 could be feasible, but more data are needed to justify such a designation. In addition, the designation of Hypersexual Disorder as primarily an Impulsive Disorder could contradict the current placement of other putatively analogous, biologically mediated appetitive behavior disorders such as Bulimia Nervosa (Eating Disorders) or Hypersomnia (Sleep Disorders). As previously stated, it is my opinion, based on the literature reviewed, that Hypersexual Disorder be considered as a Sexual Disorder associated with increased or disinhibited expressions of sexual arousal and desire in association with a dimension of impulsivity as well. (Kafka 2010, p. 393)

Kafka pointed out the central issue of the HD or CSBD diagnosis—its place within the classification of disorders and the suggestions of multiple etiologies and conceptualizations (e.g., Walton et al. 2017). His proposal of classifying hypersexuality as a disorder in the group of sexual disorders makes sense within the frame of conceptualizing sexuality along the dimensional continuum. In this concept, sexuality falls on a spectrum, with HD at one end and hyposexual desire disorder, disorder of arousal, and orgasmic disorder at the opposite end. Historically, the hypoactive end of this spectrum has been easier to define and agree upon than the hyperactive end. This has contributed significantly to the difficulty of establishing the diagnosis of HD or CSBD.

Some have suggested a more cautious approach to hypersexuality and discussed possible flaws in the concept of HD. For instance, Winters (2010) wrote that the DSM concept of mental disorder requires manifestation of a dysfunction and that the concept of HD provides no clear explanation of dysfunction. However, it is not clear whether all concepts of mental disorders include a well-defined dysfunction. Winters added that other issues with the HD diagnosis include 1) the possibility that expressed sexuality serves as a means to ameliorate the negative effect associated with some other mental disorder and is not a symptom of its own distinct disorder and 2) that if we accept that repeatedly engaging in sexual behaviors to enhance mood is symptomatic of a distinct sexual disorder, then we must accept that repetitively engaging in other, non-sexual behavior that ameliorates one's mood (e.g., shopping, exercising, hobbies) also should be pathologized but is not. Both arguments make important points, but neither is completely valid. The proposed criteria did not include anything about repeated sexual behavior enhancing mood, and some other behaviors (e.g., exercise) ameliorate the negative effects that are associated with various mental disorders. Wakefield (2012) warned of the possibility of a large number of false-positive diagnoses, "i.e., diagnoses that mistakenly label a normal variant of behavior as a mental disorder" (p. 213). He noted that some of the HD diagnostic criteria "seem to misconstrue highly culture-bound notions of morally proper sex as biological normality" and that "the evidence that normal human beings do not engage in such behavior is lacking" (p. 216). Similarly to Winters (2010), Wakefield argued that some of the HD criteria appear to pathologize adaptive behavior. These arguments, when taken individually, have some merit; however, the diagnosis of every mental disorder is a complex affair involving various criteria, distress, and other aspects considered together, not individually.

In their discussion of models explaining HD, Reid and Grant (2017) noted a lack of rigorous research to either support or refute various concepts—compulsivity, impulsivity, addiction—of hypersexual behavior. They added that researchers in fields such as addiction, compulsivity, and impulsivity do not always agree on the conceptualizations of these constructs as applied to hypersexuality (as readers of this book will come to realize after reading some of its chapters). These challenges and disagreements exist in areas of other problematic behavioral issues, such as disorders of eating, substance use, and gambling, and are even more pronounced in the area of sexuality (Reid and Grant 2017). The question is, why is sexuality—especially hypersexuality in this case—treated differently than these other behaviors? Is it a bias or an application of moral disapproval? The classification of behaviors such as addictions or substance use has also been the focus of intense debate and votes within various work groups and committees, yet we are not clear about those behaviors, either. The decision to create some descriptive diagnostic entity is more desirable and useful for further exploration than are continuous debates about which concept is more fitting.

However, in spite of the proposal from the DSM-5 Work Group on Sexual and Gender Identity Disorders and data from a field trial (Reid et al. 2012), the diagnosis of HD was not included in DSM-5, not even in Section III, "Emerging Measures and Models." The arguments against including HD, as pointed out by Kafka (2014) and others (e.g., Halperin 2011; Montgomery-Graham 2017; Moser 2011), included a lack of scientific research, inadequate neuropsychological testing, potential misuse of the diagnosis by overzealous members of the legal community, and concerns that HD should be more appropriately understood as an extension of other mental illnesses.

Some other arguments against including HD in DSM-5 are a bit puzzling. As pointed out by Kafka (2010, 2014), the number of cases of HD reported in the literature far exceeded the number of some paraphilias/paraphilic disorders, such as fetishism and frotteurism, which are both included in DSM-5. The first DSM-5 field trial for HD included 152 patients with hypersexuality (Reid et al. 2012), which is in stark contrast to the number of subjects with paraphilias included in all DSM field trials for these disorders: 3 (Blanchard 2011). Those subjects were included in the field trial for DSM-III (American Psychiatric Association 1980); there were no paraphilia trials for subsequent editions of DSM. Kafka (2014) also objected to other arguments against the HD diagnosis, such as unusually stringent requirements for the simultaneous presence of behavioral criteria and the demand for a clear categorical distinction of HD from "normal" behavior. Many psychiatric disorders have clearly dimensional characters and cannot always be distinguished from "normal" behavior at a well-defined point. He also noted that the arguments about possible misuse of the HD diagnosis in courts and forensic settings "must be resolved by applied jurisprudence as well as by refining psychiatric diagnostic criteria when indicated" (Kafka 2014, p. 1261) and not by excluding the diagnosis from classification with mental or other disorders.

In contrast to the creators of DSM-5, the ICD-11 creators erred on the side of decision rather than indecision and included hypersexuality, although under the different "label" of CSBD. In our opinion, this is an important step for patient care and for further stimulating research (Stein et al. 2020).

The decisions made by the DSM-5 and ICD-11 committees created a couple of schisms. First, the diagnosis does not exist within the framework of DSM-5 and possibly in future editions of DSM. However, a similar diagnostic construct already existed for the ICD-10, namely excessive sexual drive (F52.10). The first field trials showed that the new ICD-11 criteria work much better than the old criteria (Gaebel et al. 2020). Second, the ICD-11 classifies CSBD among the "Mental, Behavioural and Neurodevelopmental Disorders" and not among "Conditions Related to Sexual Health" (as it does sexual dysfunctions and paraphilias).

Hypersexuality and sexual compulsivity have been inundated with and besieged by myths for centuries. Do we understand them better now? Maybe. As in other fields and disciplines, attempts to define, categorize, and classify an entity are good steps forward in examining and researching it. The reality is that hypersexual behavior, whether compulsive or addictive, exists in some individuals. Another reality is that we now have some definition/diagnosis, albeit controversial, of this disordered behavior, called "compulsive sexual behavior disorder," included in the ICD. Thus, we are bringing this book to clinicians and researchers who are interested in this area and would like to better understand the concept of CSBD, further research it, and appropriately address it in their clinical practice.

REFERENCES

American Psychiatric Association: Diagnostic and Statistical Manual of Mental Disorders, 3rd Edition. Washington, DC, American Psychiatric Association, 1980

American Psychiatric Association: Diagnostic and Statistical Manual of Mental Disorders, 5th Edition. Arlington, VA, American Psychiatric Association, 2013

Blanchard R: A brief history of field trials of the DSM diagnostic criteria for paraphilias. Arch Sex Behav 40:861–862, 2011

Gaebel W, Stricker J, Riesbeck M, et al: Accuracy of diagnostic classification and clinical utility assessment of ICD-11 compared to ICD-10 in 10 mental disorders: finding from a web-based field study. Eur Arch Psychiatry Clin Neurosci 270(3):281–289, 2020

Halperin AL: The proposed diagnosis of hypersexual disorder for inclusion in DSM-5: unnecessary and harmful. Arch Sex Behav 40:487–488, 2011

Kafka MP: Hypersexual disorder: a proposed diagnosis for DSM-V. Arch Sex Behav 39(2):377–400, 2010

Kafka MP: What happened to hypersexual disorder? Arch Sex Behav 43(7):1259–1261, 2014

Montgomery-Graham S: Conceptualization and assessment of hypersexual disorder: a systematic review. Sex Med Rev 5:146–162, 2017

Moser C: Hypersexual disorder: just more muddled thinking. Arch Sex Behav 40:227–229, 231–232, 2011

Reid RC, Grant JE: In search of a parsimonious model to explain hypersexual behavior. Arch Sex Behav 46:2275–2277, 2017

Reid RC, Carpenter BN, Hook JN, et al: Report of findings in a DSM-5 field trial for hypersexual disorder. J Sex Med 9(11):2868–2877, 2012

Stein DJ, Szamari P, Gaebel W, et al: Mental, behavioral and neurodevelopmental disorders in the ICD-11: an international perspective on key changes and controversies. BMC Med 18(1):21, 2020

Wakefield JC: The DSM-5's proposed new categories of sexual disorders: the problems of false positives in sexual diagnosis. Arch Sex Behav 4:213–223, 2012

Walton MT, Cantor JM, Bhullar N, Lykins AD: Hypersexuality: a critical review and introduction to the "sexhavior cycle." Arch Sex Behav 46:2231–2251, 2017

Winters J: Hypersexual disorder: a more cautious approach. Arch Sex Behav 39:594–596, 2010

World Health Organization: International Classification of Diseases and Related Health Problems, 11th Revision. Geneva, World Health Organization, 2019

CHAPTER 2

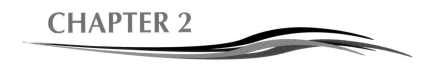

Sexual Addiction vs. CSBD

Mateusz Gola, Ph.D.
Shane W. Kraus, Ph.D.

People with compulsive sexual behavior (CSB) seek treatment for a variety of reasons. The most common reason is feeling a loss of control over the amount of time spent watching pornography (primarily via the internet), coupled most often with excessive frequency of masturbation (e.g., lapsing into a pornography spree that lasts many hours, during which the person performs multiple acts of masturbation, or, due to sudden arousal, masturbating in public restrooms or at the workplace; see Wordecha et al. 2018). Other problems related to controlling sexual behavior include the use of paid sexual services (e.g., prostitutes/escorts, massage parlors) and spending excessive amounts of money to acquire sex (Gola et al. 2016; Kor et al. 2013). Since the 1990s, scholars have debated how best to classify excessive/problematic engagement in sexual behaviors (Kraus et al. 2016) and have proposed numerous classifications, such as hypersexual disorder (HD) (Kafka 2010), impulse-control disorder (Grant et al. 2014; Kraus et al. 2018), nonparaphilic compulsive sexual behavior disorder (CSBD) (Coleman et al. 2003), behavioral addiction (Kor et al. 2013), and sexual addiction (Carnes 2013; Carnes et al. 2005, 2014). In this chapter, we review two different theoretical perspectives on describing excessive/problematic sexual behaviors: sexual addiction and CSBD.

HISTORICAL EVOLUTION OF DIAGNOSTIC CRITERIA: SEXUAL ADDICTION

One of the founding frameworks that is often used to describe excessive or problematic sexual behaviors was first introduced as "sexual addiction" by Patrick Carnes, Ph.D., in his popular book *Out of the Shadows* (Carnes 2001). He described numerous patients who sought treatment for "addictive sexual behaviors" and wrote extensively about this experience in subsequent books describing the most common symptoms of "sex addiction." According to Carnes et al. (2014), the symptoms characterizing addictive sexual behavior can be grouped into five categories:

1. Affect disturbance: Significant decrease in mood, with the possibility of depressive states or high levels of anxiety related to one's sexual behaviors and their consequences
2. Relationship disturbance: The occurrence of significant difficulties in close relationships due to one's sexual behaviors
3. Preoccupation: The occurrence of persistent, obsessive thoughts on the topic of one's sexual behaviors
4. Loss of control: Inability to stop specific sexual behaviors despite the problems and costs that are entailed
5. Associated features: For example, the experience of sexual abuse in childhood, sexual problems of one's parents, and undertaking sexual activities with minors

The sexual addiction model was proposed to follow diagnostic guidelines similar to those used for substance use disorders in DSM-5 (American Psychiatric Association 2013), in which severity is classified into three categories: mild (two or three criteria), moderate (four or five criteria), and severe (six or more criteria). The proposed criteria for sexual addiction are listed in Table 2–1.

Carnes and his colleagues developed several versions of diagnostic tests for sexual addiction (Carnes and O'Hara 1991). The Sexual Addic-

Table 2–1. Sexual addiction proposed criteria

Has repeatedly failed to resist impulses to engage in a specific sexual behavior

Has engaged in sexual behaviors to a greater extent or over a longer period than intended

Has a long-standing desire or history of unsuccessful efforts to stop, reduce, or control sexual behaviors

Spends excessive time obtaining sex, being sexual, or recovering from sexual experiences

Is obsessed with preparing for sexual activities

Frequently engages in sexual behavior when expected to be fulfilling occupational, academic, domestic, or social obligations

Continues sexual behavior despite knowing it has caused or exacerbated social, financial, psychological, or physical problems

Increases the intensity, frequency, number, or risk of sexual behaviors to achieve the desired effect, or experiences diminished effect when continuing behaviors at the same level of intensity, frequency, number, or risk

Has given up or limited social, occupational, or recreational activities because of sexual behavior

Becomes upset, anxious, restless, or irritable if unable to engage in sexual behavior

Severity: mild (two or three criteria), moderate (four or five criteria) and severe (six or more criteria)

tion Screening Test–Revised (SAST-R; Carnes et al. 2010), next to the Hypersexual Behavior Inventory (Reid et al. 2011), is the most popular measure of total symptoms of sexual addiction. This 45-item measure includes 20 core items to assess sexual addiction. An additional four subscales (Internet, Men's, Women's, and Gay Men's) assess specific problems of sexual addiction for certain groups (Carnes et al. 2010).

A shorter version of the SAST was developed as the six-item PATHOS questionnaire (Carnes et al. 2012). This brief questionnaire measures six domains of purported relevance in sexual addiction (i.e., Preoccupied, Ashamed, Treatment, Hurts others, Out of control, Sad). In Carnes et al.'s (2012) initial paper, items were evaluated with both inpatients and outpatients who were seeking treatment for sexual addiction. Using a cutoff score of 3, the PATHOS demonstrated acceptable sensitivity and specificity distinguishing between the control group and treatment-seeking patients (Carnes et al. 2012).

Thus far, the SAST and PATHOS have been validated in international samples from Poland (Gola et al. 2017a), Spain (Castro-Calvo et al. 2018),

Nigeria (Abdullahi and Udofia 2015), and Belgium (Wéry et al. 2016). Despite its popular use in research studies, the sexual addiction framework first proposed by Carnes and his colleagues has not been widely adopted, nor was it considered for DSM-5.

HD, proposed by Kafka (2010), evolved in the 2010s to describe clinical hypersexuality (hypersexual behaviors) among treatment-seeking patients (Reid et al. 2012). HD was first proposed by the DSM-5 Work Group on Sexual and Gender Identity Disorders for inclusion among the sexual dysfunctions. The Work Group described HD as a persistent pattern of behavior involving intense preoccupation with sexual fantasies, urges, and behaviors that causes adverse consequences and clinically significant distress or impairment in social, occupational, or other important areas of functioning (Kafka 2010). Despite strong findings from a field trial (Reid et al. 2012), the proposed disorder was ultimately rejected by the DSM-5 Task Force. Specifically, the Task Force raised concerns about the lack of a robust research base across areas such as structural and functional brain imaging, molecular genetics, pathophysiology, epidemiology, and neuropsychological testing (Piquet-Pessôa et al. 2014). Concerns were also raised about the possible forensic misuse of the category for civil commitment of U.S. sex offenders (Reid and Kafka 2014). In 2019, CSBD was formally included in the ICD-11 to describe excessive/problematic sexual behaviors (Kraus et al. 2018; World Health Organization 2019).

OVERVIEW OF CSBD

The ICD-11 Working Group on Obsessive-Compulsive and Related Disorders proposed a conceptualization of impulse-control disorders as the repeated failure to resist an impulse, drive, or urge to engage in a behavior that is rewarding to the person, at least initially, despite long-term harm (Kraus et al. 2018). The Working Group recommended that a category of "compulsive sexual behavior disorder" be included in this grouping (Grant et al. 2014) because it emphasized that sexual behaviors shared a commonality with other disorders involving difficulty with impulse regulation. Despite concerns about the potential for misuse of this category to label nonpathological sexual behavior, the Working Group decided that there was substantial scientific basis for adding CSBD to the ICD-11. More importantly, including CSBD in the ICD-11 would provide needed guidance for improving and standardizing the identification of this condition and facilitating appropriate treatment for affected persons around the world (Kraus et al. 2018). The World Health

---

Table 2–2.   ICD-11 diagnostic criteria for compulsive sexual behavior disorder

---

Essential (required) features for compulsive sexual behavior disorder:

A persistent pattern of failure to control intense, repetitive sexual impulses or urges resulting in repetitive sexual behavior, must be manifested in one or more of the following:

1a. Engaging in repetitive sexual activities has become a central focus of the person's life to the point of neglecting health and personal care or other interests, activities, and responsibilities (yes/no).

1b. The person has made numerous unsuccessful efforts to control or significantly reduce repetitive sexual behavior (yes/no)

1c. The person continues to engage in repetitive sexual behavior despite adverse consequences (e.g., repeated relationship disruption, occupational consequences, negative impact on health) (yes/no).

1d. The person continues to engage in repetitive sexual behavior even when the individual derives little or no satisfaction from it (yes/no).

2. The pattern of failure to control intense, sexual impulses or urges and resulting repetitive sexual behavior is manifested over an extended period (e.g., 6 months or more) (must be met).

3. The pattern of repetitive sexual behavior causes marked distress or significant impairment in personal, family, social, educational, occupational, or other important areas of functioning (Must be met). *Note for rule out:* Distress that is entirely related to moral judgments and disapproval about sexual impulses, urges, or behaviors is not enough to meet this requirement.

Source.   World Health Organization 2019.

Organization Secretariat approved the inclusion of CSBD (code 6C72) in the ICD-11 in June 2019.

The essential features of CSBD are similar to criteria in highlighting the core clinical characteristics of the condition, but they are meant to be less rigid because they rely less on arbitrary cutoffs or symptom counts and are intended to support the exercise of clinical judgment in assigning the diagnosis to treatment-seeking patients (First et al. 2015). The ICD-11 diagnostic criteria for CSBD are listed in Table 2–2.

The diagnostic guidelines for CSBD emphasize that the diagnosis should be applied to a pattern of sexual behavior only when the person exhibits a persistent failure to control intense, repetitive sexual impulses or urges that lead to CSB, manifested in specific outcomes and associated with distress or functional impairment, for a period of 6 months or longer. The diagnosis should not be given in the absence of marked distress or significant impairment or if the person's distress is entirely related to moral judgments and disapproval of sexual impulses, urges, or behaviors. The long duration requirement (≥6 months) is intended to avoid application of the diagnosis to briefer periods of time in which increased sexual activity could be better explained by relationship changes, environmental factors, or the adverse effects of medication.

Mr. G

Mr. G is a heterosexual married male in his early 30s with a history of depression who self-identified as "addicted to porn" and sought treatment at an outpatient clinic. He denied any substance use. He reported that he began using pornography regularly in his early teenage years and had engaged in frequent masturbation to pornography for the past 10 years, viewing pornography for longer periods of time when his wife traveled for work (which often occurred monthly). When his wife was away, he would view pornography daily, often several times a day. He described "porn binges" that consisted of heavy pornography viewing (≥4 hours) accompanied by repeated masturbation. He reported satisfactory sexual activity with his wife, although he thought his pornography use was interfering with their intimacy and relationship because it consumed his thoughts throughout the day. He described these thoughts as intrusive and his pornography use as compulsive, and he gained little to no satisfaction from it. He reported frequent unsuccessful attempts to quit viewing pornography and intense urges to view pornography after several days of deprivation.

The Compulsive Sexual Behavior Inventory (CSBI-13) is a 13-item screening tool developed to assesses the core feature of CSBD: functional impairment or distress associated with difficulty controlling one's sexual feelings, urges, and behaviors (Coleman et al. 2020). The CSBI-13 has shown adequate reliability, criterion validity, and discriminant and convergent validity (Miner et al. 2017). Recently, Böthe et al. (2020) developed the Compulsive Sexual Behavior Disorder–19 (CSBD-19) as a short, valid, and reliable measure of CSBD symptoms based on ICD-11 diagnostic guidelines. Further research is needed to develop and validate clinical measures that can accurately diagnose patients with CSBD. This is particularly relevant because the nature and frequency of individuals' sexual behaviors vary substantially (Laumann et al. 1994), and it is important to distinguish factors such as high levels of sexual activity due to a high sexual drive from loss of control over one's sexual behavior in ways that produce distress and functional impairment. More research is also needed to examine sex differences in CSBD diagnostic criteria as well as to explore possible cultural, ethnic, and sexual minority group differences (Kowalewska et al. 2020).

COMPULSIVE SEXUAL BEHAVIOR AS AN IMPULSE-CONTROL DISORDER

It is difficult to draw a clear line between addiction, impulse-control disorder, and compulsion because these concepts overlap: impulses or urges to engage in repetitive behaviors are core features of addiction. They are distinctive in that addiction is typically associated with additional features, including tolerance and withdrawal, whereas for impulse-control disorders, such as kleptomania and pyromania, the pathology is assumed to lie primarily within the person. However, due to the recent extension of the term *addiction* to include behavioral addictions such as gambling (in DSM-5) or gaming (in ICD-11), even withdrawal symptoms are no longer universal. Individuals with CSB in some studies exhibit significantly higher levels of impulsiveness than do control subjects (Antons and Brand 2018; Mechelmans et al. 2014; Miner et al. 2009), although similar associations have been observed in people addicted to gambling (Specker et al. 1995), alcohol (Lejoyeux et al. 1999), or cocaine (Li et al. 2008). One could say that impulsivity as a character trait (perhaps via neurobiological mechanisms) predisposes to addiction, although it is not a necessary condition, because some people with addictions have low impulsivity (Gola et al. 2017b; Li et al. 2009). Some studies of patients with CSBD show no difference from healthy control subjects in terms of general impulsivity but very specific increased sensitivity for erotic cues among those with CSBD (Gola et al. 2017b). Such increased sensitivity toward one category of cues is typical for addiction and has been described in detail by incentive salience theory as a main factor underlying craving in addiction (Olney et al. 2018; Robinson and Berridge 1993). Higher susceptibility for development of this neural mechanism has been linked to specific genetic factors (Forbes et al. 2009; Gola et al. 2015), but this has not yet been studied in CSBD. Therefore, it is suggested that impulse-control disorder as a broad category that stresses the impulsive character of actions is a good starting place for CSBD given the current stage of knowledge.

Precise prevalence estimates of CSBD among clinical and nonclinical populations remain elusive (Gola and Potenza 2018; Kraus et al. 2016). A recent study of 2,325 U.S. adults found that 8.6% of the representative sample (7.0% of females and 10.3% of males) endorsed clinically relevant levels of distress or impairment associated with concerns about sexual feelings, urges, and behaviors (Dickenson et al. 2018). Specific to pornography use, data from a U.S. nationally representative sample of 2,075 internet users found that approximately half of the sample ($n = 1,056$) reported past-year use of pornography, and 11% of male and 3% of female subjects reported "feeling addicted to pornography" (Grubbs et al. 2019). Among persons seeking treatment for CSBD and hypersexuality, most individuals (>80%) reported concerns with pornography use (Gola and Draps 2018; Kraus et al. 2015; Reid et al. 2012; Scanavino et al. 2013). Differences may also exist between individuals who predominantly engage in online behaviors and those whose behavior involves physical proximity and contact.

Males exhibit CSB more frequently than females (Kafka 2010; Lewczuk et al. 2017), although robust data examining gender differences are lacking. Additionally, higher rates have been noted among individuals with substance use disorders (Stavro et al. 2013). Among those who seek treatment, CSB negatively impacts occupational, relationship, physical health, and mental health functioning (Reid et al. 2012). However, systematic data are lacking regarding its prevalence across different populations and any associated sociocultural and sociodemographic factors, including among individuals who do not seek treatment (Gola and Potenza 2018).

Rates of co-occurrence are elevated between CSB and mood, substance use, and personality disorders (Kraus et al. 2015; Raymond et al. 2003). CSB is also positively associated with sexual risk taking, such as sexual intercourse without condoms, among both heterosexual and non-heterosexual persons and elevated rates of HIV and other sexually transmitted infections (Yoon et al. 2016). For example, in a recent study of 119 HIV-infected males, Chumakov et al. (2019) found that 29.5% of men who have sex with men and 12.1% of men who have sex with women had CSB. Recent evidence also suggests that suicide risk is higher among individuals with CSB compared with those without CSB (Kraus et al. 2017; Scanavino et al. 2013). More research examining the clinical and medical complications associated with CSB among clinical populations is needed.

CSB is associated with elevated self-reported impulsivity, which is relevant across both impulse-control disorders and disorders of addiction, although laboratory-based measures have not yet explored this in depth. Most neurobiological studies have focused on online pornography use rather than other sexual behaviors. A recent review of neuroimaging studies found that CSB was associated with altered functioning in brain regions and networks implicated in sensitization, habituation, diminished impulse control, and reward processing in patterns such as substance, gambling, and gaming addictions (Gola and Draps 2018; Kowalewska et al. 2018; Stark et al. 2018). However, whether these same patterns are also present in other ICDs remains to be investigated.

Dopamine replacement therapies used for patients with Parkinson's disease have sometimes resulted in patterns of impulse-control problems that resemble CSBD (Weintraub et al. 2010). The possible efficacy of naltrexone in reducing urges and behaviors associated with CSBD has also been noted (Kraus et al. 2015; Raymond et al. 2002), providing some evidence for opioid-related modulation of dopaminergic activity in mesolimbic pathways in CSBD. Therapy with selective serotonin reuptake inhibitors also seems to be helpful for CSBD symptom reduction (Gola and Potenza 2016). A useful focus for future neuroimaging studies would be craving and urge states that may precede both compulsive behaviors and substance use among individuals with substance dependence.

SUMMARY

The history of conceptualizing out-of-control sexual behaviors (from addiction, through hypersexual behavior disorder, to CSBD being recognized by the World Health Organization in ICD-11) and the variety of proposed criteria show how complex this clinical phenomenon is and how our understanding of it has evolved (see Grubbs et al. 2020 for discussion). Examples discussed in this chapter, together with results of recent psychological, behavioral, and neuroimaging studies, suggest that many individuals meeting CSBD criteria share similar characteristics with those who have behavioral or substance addiction. However, not all people who manifest out-of-control sexual behavior are indeed addicted to sexual activity (either involving others or solitary with pornography). A similar set of symptoms may be caused by anxiety disorders, levodopa overdose (Gola and Potenza 2016), mania, disinhibition (e.g., in advanced dementia; Miller et al. 1986), or general impulse-control issues.

A person's sense of losing control over sexual behavior can result from a variety of social and cultural factors interacting with specific psychological characteristics. For example, someone raised in a conservative environment with moral and cultural beliefs that disapprove of premarital interpersonal or solitary sexual activity may experience significant discomfort from any sexual arousal that comes from visual erotic stimulation, whether via the internet or in a new environment, such as moving to college (Efrati and Mikulincer 2018; Grubbs et al. 2019). On the other hand, there are large groups of people who express high sexual activity (or frequent pornography use) and experience no negative consequences (Gola et al. 2016). Thus, it is important to examine the source of a person's discomfort about sexual activity and keep in mind that mere quantitative aspects of individual sexual activities—as long as they are not a source of suffering for that person or others—should not be labeled too readily in terms of what is "normal" and what is pathological. The data presented here should be considered evidence for the claim that out-of-control sexual behavior is a complex and heterogeneous set of disorders that—similarities at the level of symptoms notwithstanding—have different mechanisms. The aims and methods of effective therapeutic intervention should take these mechanisms into account, and future studies will need to consider rapidly changing technologies that provide new forms of potentially problematic sexual behaviors (e.g., sexting, one-night-stand dating, and pornography use, including immersive and tactile technologies) that may result in new categories of symptoms. We suspect that excessive/problematic sexual behaviors will mirror ever-changing technologies, particularly where access to new sexual partners or visually stimulating material has been facilitated via the internet.

In our opinion, the World Health Organization's decision to name this new clinical entity describing out-of-control sexual behaviors as *compulsive* sexual behavior disorder and to place it within the category of *impulse*-control disorders with diagnostic criteria that share most of the features of *addictions* is a good compromise, taking into account the current state of rapidly developing knowledge on this topic and all previous concerns, together with future challenges.

REFERENCES

Abdullahi H, Udofia O: A pilot psychometric investigation of the Sexual Addiction Screening Test (SAST) and Women's Sexual Addiction Screening Test (W-SAST) in a Nigerian hospital setting. Sexual Addiction and Compulsivity 22(1):16–25, 2015

American Psychiatric Association: Diagnostic and Statistical Manual of Mental Disorders, 5th Edition. Arlington, VA, American Psychiatric Association, 2013

Antons S, Brand M: Trait and state impulsivity in males with tendency towards Internet-pornography-use disorder. Addict Behav 79:171–177, 2018

Böthe B, Potenza MN, Griffiths MD, et al: The development of the Compulsive Sexual Behavior Disorder Scale (CSBD-19): an ICD-11 based screening measure across three languages. J Behav Addict 9(2):247–258, 2020

Carnes P: Out of the Shadows: Understanding Sexual Addiction. Center City, MN, Hazelden, 2001

Carnes P: Don't Call It Love: Recovery From Sexual Addiction. New York, Bantam, 2013

Carnes P, O'Hara S: Sexual Addiction Screening Test (SAST). Tennessee Nurse 54(3):29, 1991

Carnes PJ, Murray RE, Charpentier L: Bargains with chaos: sex addicts and addiction interaction disorder. Sexual Addiction and Compulsivity 12(2–3):79–120, 2005

Carnes P, Green B, Carnes S: The same yet different: refocusing the Sexual Addiction Screening Test (SAST) to reflect orientation and gender. Sexual Addiction and Compulsivity 17(1):7–30, 2010

Carnes PJ, Green BA, Merlo LJ, et al: PATHOS: a brief screening application for assessing sexual addiction. J Addict Med 6(1):29–34, 2012

Carnes PJ, Hopkins TA, Green BA: Clinical relevance of the proposed sexual addiction diagnostic criteria: relation to the Sexual Addiction Screening Test–Revised. J Addict Med 8(6):450–461, 2014

Castro-Calvo J, Ballester-Arnal R, Billieux J, et al: Spanish validation of the Sexual Addiction Screening Test. J Behav Addict 7(3):584–600, 2018

Chumakov EM, Petrova NN, Kraus SW: Compulsive sexual behavior in HIV-infected men in a community based sample, Russia. Sexual Addiction and Compulsivity 26(1–2):164–175, 2019

Coleman E, Raymond N, McBean A: Assessment and treatment of compulsive sexual behavior. Minn Med 86(7):42–47, 2003

Coleman E, Swinburne Romine R, Dickenson J, Miner MH: Compulsive Sexual Behavior Inventory–13, in Handbook of Sexuality-Related Measures, 4th Edition. Edited by Milhausen RR, Sakaluk JK, Fisher TD, et al. New York, Routledge, 2020

Dickenson JA, Gleason N, Coleman E, Miner MH: Prevalence of distress associated with difficulty controlling sexual urges, feelings, and behaviors in the United States. JAMA Network Open 1(7):e184468, 2018

Efrati Y, Mikulincer M: Individual-based Compulsive Sexual Behavior Scale: its development and importance in examining compulsive sexual behavior. J Sex Marital Ther 44(3):249–259, 2018

First MB, Reed GM, Hyman SE, Saxena S: The development of the ICD-11 clinical descriptions and diagnostic guidelines for mental and behavioural disorders. World Psychiatry 14(1):82–90, 2015

Forbes EE, Brown SM, Kimak M, et al: Genetic variation in components of dopamine neurotransmission impacts ventral striatal reactivity associated with impulsivity. Mol Psychiatry 14(1):60–70, 2009

Gola M, Draps M: Ventral striatal reactivity in compulsive sexual behaviors. Front Psychiatry 9:546, 2018

Gola M, Potenza MN: Paroxetine treatment of problematic pornography use: a case series. J Behav Addict 5(3):529–532, 2016

Gola M, Potenza MN: The proof of the pudding is in the tasting: data are needed to test models and hypotheses related to compulsive sexual behaviors. Arch Sex Behav 47(5):1323–1325, 2018

Gola M, Miyakoshi M, Sescousse G: Sex, impulsivity, and anxiety: interplay between ventral striatum and amygdala reactivity in sexual behaviors. J Neurosci 35(46):15227–15229, 2015

Gola M, Lewczuk K, Skorko M: What matters: quantity or quality of pornography use? Psychological and behavioral factors of seeking treatment for problematic pornography use. J Sex Med 13(5):815–824, 2016

Gola M, Skorko M, Kowalewska E, et al: Polish adaptation of Sexual Addiction Screening Test–Revised (SAST-PL-M). Polish Psychiatry 51(1):95–115, 2017a

Gola M, Wordecha M, Sescousse G, et al: Can pornography be addictive? An fMRI study of men seeking treatment for problematic pornography use. Neuropsychopharmacology 42(10):2021–2031, 2017b

Grant JE, Atmaca M, Fineberg NA, et al: Impulse control disorders and "behavioural addictions" in the ICD-11. World Psychiatry 13(2):125–127, 2014

Grubbs JB, Kraus SW, Perry SL: Self-reported addiction to pornography in a nationally representative sample: the roles of use habits, religiousness, and moral incongruence. J Behav Addict 8(1):88–93, 2019

Grubbs JB, Grant JT, Lee BN, et al: Sexual addiction 25 years on: a systematic and methodological review of empirical literature and an agenda for future research. Clin Psychol Rev 82:101925, 2020

Kafka MP: Hypersexual disorder: a proposed diagnosis for DSM-V. Arch Sex Behav 39(2):377–400, 2010

Kor A, Fogel YA, Reid RC, Potenza MN: Should hypersexual disorder be classified as an addiction? Sexual Addiction and Compulsivity 20(1–2):27–47, 2013

Kowalewska E, Grubbs JB, Potenza MN, et al: Neurocognitive mechanisms in compulsive sexual behavior disorder. Curr Sex Health Rep 10(4):255–264, 2018

Kowalewska E, Gola M, Kraus SW, Lew-Starowicz M: Spotlight on compulsive sexual behavior disorder: a systematic review of research on women. Neuropsychiatr Dis Treat 16:2025–2043, 2020

Kraus SW, Potenza MN, Martino S, Grant JE: Examining the psychometric properties of the Yale-Brown Obsessive-Compulsive Scale in a sample of compulsive pornography users. Compr Psychiatry 59:117–122, 2015

Kraus SW, Voon V, Potenza MN: Should compulsive sexual behavior be considered an addiction? Addiction 111(12):2097–2106, 2016

Kraus SW, Martino S, Potenza MN, et al: Examining compulsive sexual behavior and psychopathology among a sample of postdeployment U.S. male and female military veterans. Mil Psychol 29(2):143–156, 2017

Kraus SW, Krueger RB, Briken P, et al: Compulsive sexual behaviour disorder in the ICD-11. World Psychiatry 17(1):109–110, 2018

Laumann EO, Gagnon JH, Michael RT, Michaels S: The Social Organization of Sexuality: Sexual Practices in the United States. Chicago, IL, University of Chicago, 1994

Lejoyeux M, Feuché N, Loi S, et al: Study of impulse-control disorders among alcohol-dependent patients. J Clin Psychiatry 60(5):302–305, 1999

Lewczuk K, Szmyd J, Skorko M, Gola M: Treatment seeking for problematic pornography use among women. J Behav Addict 6(4):445–456, 2017

Li CSR, Huang C, Yan P, et al: Neural correlates of impulse control during stop signal inhibition in cocaine-dependent men. Neuropsychopharmacology 33(8):1798–1806, 2008

Li CSR, Luo X, Yan P, et al: Altered impulse control in alcohol dependence: neural measures of stop signal performance. Alcohol Clin Exp Res 33(4):740–750, 2009

Mechelmans DJ, Irvine M, Banca P, et al: Enhanced attentional bias towards sexually explicit cues in individuals with and without compulsive sexual behaviours. PLoS One 9(8):e105476, 2014

Miller BL, Cummings JL, McIntyre H, et al: Hypersexuality or altered sexual preference following brain injury. J Neurol Neurosurg Psychiatry 49(8):867–873, 1986

Miner MH, Raymond N, Mueller BA, et al: Preliminary investigation of the impulsive and neuroanatomical characteristics of compulsive sexual behavior. Psychiatry Res 174(2):146–151, 2009

Miner MH, Raymond N, Coleman E, Romine RS: Investigating clinically and scientifically useful cut points on the Compulsive Sexual Behavior Inventory. J Sex Med 14(5):715–720, 2017

Olney N, Wertz T, LaPorta Z, et al: Comparison of acute physiological and psychological responses between moderate-intensity continuous exercise and three regimes of high-intensity interval training. J Strength Cond Res 32(8):2130–2138, 2018

Piquet-Pessôa M, Ferreira GM, Melca IA, Fontenelle LF: DSM-5 and the decision not to include sex, shopping or stealing as addictions. Curr Addict Rep 1(3):172–176, 2014

Raymond NC, Grant JE, Kim SW, Coleman E: Treatment of compulsive sexual behaviour with naltrexone and serotonin reuptake inhibitors: two case studies. Int Clin Psychopharmacol 17(4):201–205, 2002

Raymond NC, Coleman E, Miner MH: Psychiatric comorbidity and compulsive/impulsive traits in compulsive sexual behavior. Compr Psychiatry 44(5):370–380, 2003

Reid RC, Kafka MP: Controversies about hypersexual disorder and the DSM-5. Curr Sex Health Rep 6(4):259–264, 2014

Reid RC, Garos S, Carpenter BN: Reliability, validity, and psychometric development of the Hypersexual Behavior Inventory in an outpatient sample of men. Sexual Addiction and Compulsivity 18(1):30–51, 2011

Reid RC, Carpenter BN, Hook JN, et al: Report of findings in a DSM-5 field trial for hypersexual disorder. J Sex Med 9(11):2868–2877, 2012

Robinson TE, Berridge KC: The neural basis of drug craving: an incentive-sensitization theory of addiction. Brain Res Rev 18(3):247–291, 1993

Scanavino MdT, Ventuneac A, Abdo CHN, et al: Compulsive sexual behavior and psychopathology among treatment-seeking men in São Paulo, Brazil. Psychiatry Res 209(3):518–524, 2013

Specker SM, Carlson GA, Christenson GA, Marcotte M: Impulse control disorders and attention deficit disorder in pathological gamblers. Ann Clin Psychiatry 7(4):175–179, 1995

Stark R, Klucken T, Potenza MN, et al: A current understanding of the behavioral neuroscience of compulsive sexual behavior disorder and problematic pornography use. Curr Behav Neurosci Rep 5(4):218–231, 2018

Stavro K, Rizkallah E, Dinh-Williams L, et al: Hypersexuality among a substance use disorder population. Sexual Addiction and Compulsivity 20(3):210–216, 2013

Weintraub D, Koester J, Potenza MN, et al: Impulse control disorders in Parkinson disease: a cross-sectional study of 3090 patients. Arch Neurol 67(5):589–595, 2010

Wéry A, Burnay J, Karila L, Billieux J: The Short French Internet Addiction Test adapted to online sexual activities: validation and links with online sexual preferences and addiction symptoms. J Sex Res 53(6):701–710, 2016

Wordecha M, Wilk M, Kowalewska E, et al: "Pornographic binges" as a key characteristic of males seeking treatment for compulsive sexual behaviors: qualitative and quantitative 10-week-long diary assessment. J Behav Addict 7(2):433–444, 2018

World Health Organization: International Classification of Diseases and Related Health Problems, 11th Revision. Geneva, World Health Organization, 2019

Yoon IS, Houang ST, Hirshfield S, Downing MJ: Compulsive sexual behavior
    and HIV/STI risk: a review of current literature. Curr Addict Rep 3(4):387–
    399, 2016

CHAPTER 3

Compulsive Sexual Behavior and Substance Use Disorders

Shane W. Kraus, Ph.D.

Ami Popat-Jain, Ph.D.

Marc N. Potenza, M.D., Ph.D.

The precise rates of compulsive sexual behavior (CSB) among individuals with substance use disorders (SUDs) are evolving. However, at this time, preliminary data collected from clinical and nonclinical samples suggest high overlapping rates between both conditions. This chapter examines the associations between CSB and SUDs and other addictive disorders, including gambling disorder.

Overall, we found high rates of CSB among individuals with SUDs, particularly in regard to alcohol, opioid, and stimulant use disorders.

This appeared most pronounced among specific groups, such as men who have sex with men, U.S. military veterans, and individuals seeking residential treatment. Gambling disorder (including subthreshold at-risk or problem gambling) often co-occurs with CSB, although rates appear to be lower (<20%) compared with SUDs. Associations between CSB and cannabis use remain understudied, but preliminary data suggest cannabis is positively associated with increased sexual risk taking. Given the high rates of CSB among those with SUDs, we recommend therapeutic modalities developed to address both behaviors concurrently. Currently, several types of interventions have demonstrated positive outcomes, including psychotherapies such as cognitive-behavioral therapy, acceptance and commitment therapy (ACT), and mindfulness-based interventions, although more information testing the efficacy and effectiveness of treatments is needed. Lastly, more research is needed to study CSB and addictive disorders in diverse populations (e.g., those who identify as female, persons of color), because much of the current research is based predominantly on European/white male samples.

COMPULSIVE SEXUAL BEHAVIOR

Historically, CSBs have been called by various names. The lack of consensus around the definition of compulsive sexual behavior disorder (CSBD) and the names for types and patterns of CSBs more broadly has arguably created confusion and slowed research efforts (Kuzma and Black 2008). Prevalence estimates of CSBD remain elusive given current gaps in the literature (Gola and Potenza 2018; Kraus et al. 2016), with some estimating rates between 3% and 5% for the general population (Kafka 2010). In a study of 2,108 U.S. university students, 3% of male and 1% of female students reported symptoms consistent with CSBD (Odlaug et al. 2013). A more recent study of 2,325 adults in the United States found that 8.6% of the representative sample (7.0% of females and 10.3% of males) endorsed clinically relevant levels of distress or impairment associated with difficulty controlling sexual feelings, urges, and behaviors (Dickenson et al. 2018). *Sexual impulsivity*, defined as "a tendency to engage in sexual behaviors quickly or without fully thinking through the consequences," was acknowledged in a national sample of 34,653 U.S. adults by 14.7% of subjects (18.9% of males and 10.9% of females) and was associated with multiple mood, anxiety, substance use, and personality disorders (Erez et al. 2014). As such, CSBs may be more prevalent than previously reported. Further research is needed to accurately obtain prevalence rates in the general and clinical populations.

Most studies of CSBD, especially of forms such as problematic pornography use, have predominantly or solely involved men. However, some studies have investigated CSBs in women. In a nonclinical sample, women who had symptoms of psychosis and elevated impulsivity (related to motor and planning) may have been at greater risk for experiencing sexual compulsivity (Carvalho et al. 2015). Among women in a residential treatment program, those who were less likely to engage in mindfulness-based behaviors were more likely to experience both SUDs and CSBs (Brem et al. 2017b). These findings suggest that women who are at elevated risk for addictive behaviors and CSB may benefit from mindfulness-based treatment. Erez et al. (2014) evaluated gender-related differences in the co-occurrence of sexual impulsivity and mental illness. Sexual impulsivity was associated with multiple psychiatric disorders for both men and women. Although sexual impulsivity was more often reported by men, relationships between sexual impulsivity and psychopathology—particularly with respect to alcohol use disorders, phobias, and multiple personality disorders (particularly Cluster B)—were stronger in women than in men.

In this chapter, problematic sexual behavior (e.g., hypersexuality, sexual addiction) is referred to as *compulsive sexual behavior* (CSB). During the considerations for DSM-5 (American Psychiatric Association 2013), hypersexual disorder (HD) was defined and studied but was ultimately not included in the manual (Kafka 2010). CSBD recently has been included in the ICD-11 (World Health Organization 2019).

SUBSTANCE USE DISORDERS: PREVALENCE AND CORRELATES

Black et al. (1997) examined rates of psychopathology in 36 patients reporting issues with CSBs. Rates of substance use were particularly high; specifically, the authors found a 6-month prevalence of around 19% for alcohol abuse or dependence (58% lifetime), 3% for drug abuse or dependence (33% lifetime), and 22% for any SUD (64% lifetime). Researchers (Kafka and Hennen 2002) studying psychopathology among 120 male patients with paraphilias and related disorders (a disorder construct very similar to CSBD) also found high rates of mood (71.6%), anxiety (38.3%), and substance use (40.8%) disorders, most of which were characterized by alcohol (30.0%), cocaine (14.1%), or cannabis (18.3%) use disorders. Similarly, Raymond et al. (2003) found that roughly one-third (29%) of 29 patients with CSB also met criteria for SUDs (e.g., 21% alcohol, 8% cannabis, 4% cocaine), and the percentage jumped to 71% for lifetime histories (e.g., 63% alcohol, 38% cannabis, 13% cocaine).

Carnes et al. (2005) examined addictions in 894 men and 588 women seeking treatment for "sexual addiction." Among men, co-occurring addictive behaviors included alcohol use disorder (45.8%), substance abuse (40.1%), compulsive eating (17.6%), and compulsive gambling (8.2%). Among women, co-occurring addictive behaviors included alcohol use disorder (45.9%), substance abuse (40.8%), compulsive eating (33.88%), and compulsive gambling (4.2%). Together, these data suggest frequent co-occurrences between CSBs and addictive behaviors and disorders. Among 211 Canadian patients seeking treatment for SUDs, Stavro et al. (2013) found that 25% of the participants screened positive (score ≥53) on the Sexual Addiction Screening Test–Revised (SAST-R), a measure of sexual addiction (Carnes et al. 2010). Furthermore, they found that a positive screen on the SAST-R was associated with self-reported male gender and cocaine abuse/dependence.

Among 86 Brazilian men with CSB, Scanavino et al. (2013) found relatively low rates of substance use: alcohol dependence (5.8%) and substance dependence (7.0%). In a larger study of Croatian men (N=1,998), one subset was classified as hypersexual (n=57) (Štulhofer et al. 2016). Among this group, hypersexuality was associated with being single, not exclusively heterosexual, religious, depressed, prone to sexual boredom, experiencing substance abuse consequences, holding negative attitudes toward pornography use, and evaluating one's sexual morality more negatively. Moreover, hypersexual men were 1.8 times more likely to report consequences from substance abuse (alcohol or drug) compared with nonhypersexual men (Štulhofer et al. 2016). Another study by Farré et al. (2015) compared substance use in 59 patients with sexual addiction with 2,190 patients with gambling disorder. They found similar rates of tobacco use (gambling disorder 22.7% vs. sexual addiction 17.7%) and alcohol abuse (gambling disorder 14.9% vs. sexual addiction 14.0%) but higher other-drug use among patients with sexual addiction (21.8%) compared with patients with gambling disorder (9.7%). Their results highlight the high co-occurrence of behavioral and substance addictions among people with gambling disorder and CSB.

Elmquist et al. (2016) studied the clinical characteristics of 349 male patients seeking treatment for SUDs. Most were diagnosed with alcohol dependence (59.8%) as their primary substance use disorder, followed by opioid dependence (18.3%), cannabis abuse (2.7%), polysubstance dependence (2.4%), and amphetamine dependence (2.4%). Alcohol use severity, but not drug use severity, was positively correlated with CSB. In another study of 150 men being treated for SUDs (Brem et al. 2017a), researchers examined experiential avoidance (defined as attempts to avoid thoughts, feelings, memories, physical sensations, or internal experiences) as one potential mechanism underlying the relation between men's symptoms of depression and anxiety and their CSBs. Positive bivariate associations were also noted between CSB and alcohol use severity but not drug use severity. Furthermore, researchers found that experiential avoidance explains the relationship between both depression and anxiety symptoms and CSBs among men in residential substance use treatment (Brem et al. 2017a).

In another study (Shorey et al. 2016), researchers studied the medical records of 271 male patients seeking treatment for alcohol and drug use problems. Study participants completed self-report measures on alcohol and drug use, dispositional mindfulness, and CSB. Bivariate correlations found that dispositional mindfulness was negatively associated with CSB. After adjusting for alcohol and drug use and problems in hierarchical regression analyses, dispositional mindfulness remained negatively associated with CSB among these men.

Brem et al. (2018) examined experiential avoidance as a mediator of the relationship between defectiveness/shame beliefs, PTSD symptoms, and CSB in 446 women with SUDs. CSB was positively correlated with alcohol use and drug use severity as well as PTSD symptoms and feelings of defectiveness/shame. Results revealed that experiential avoidance partially mediated the relationship between both PTSD symptoms and defectiveness/shame beliefs and CSB. Moreover, the authors posited that targeting experiential avoidance among women with comorbid SUDs and CSB may be beneficial for enhanced treatment outcomes.

In 485 patients receiving treatment for SUDs, researchers (Deneke et al. 2015) examined the prevalence of at-risk sexual addiction (SAST-R score ≥6) and other co-occurring psychiatric disorders across three programs (30-day primary care, 30-day relapse, and 9-day extended). Prevalence estimates for at-risk sexual addiction by unit were primary care 18%, relapse 18.6%, and extended care 29.0%. No differences for substance use were noted between low-risk (n=383) and at-risk (n=102) groups for use of alcohol (74.7% vs. 79.4%), opioids (36% vs. 32.4%), sedatives (27.4% vs. 22.5%), or inhalants (10.2% vs. 7.8%). However, significant differences were observed in substance use between the low-risk and at-risk groups for use of cannabis (17% vs. 35.3%), cocaine (17% vs. 27.5%), or amphetamines (8.9% vs. 23.5%). The authors also found significant differences in psychiatric disorders between the low-risk and at-risk groups for mood disorders (10.4% vs. 25.5%), PTSD (7% vs. 13.7%), or impulse-control disorders (1.6% vs. 11.8%) (Deneke et al. 2015). Lastly, researchers (Diehl et al. 2019) examined the frequency of early maltreatment experiences and adult sexual trauma among 134 Brazilian adults seeking treatment for SUDs. They found that one-third of drug users who reported physical abuse in childhood screened positive for sexual addiction (SAST score ≤6). In summary, there is a high co-occurrence between CSB and SUDs among treatment-seeking and community-based samples.

Cannabis

Research has found relationships between CSB or sexual risk behavior and cannabis use. In one study, adolescent males who were actively using marijuana more frequently reported risky sexual behavior (Dembo et al. 2014). Another study found that adolescents were more likely to engage in risky sexual behavior, specifically involving less use of condoms, when using marijuana (Bryan et al. 2012). In 120 Nigerian adults (62% male), researchers examined associations between depression, sexual compulsivity, and sexual risk behaviors. Among cannabis-using adults, sexual compulsivity was significantly associated with female gender, age at first cannabis use, self-esteem, and sexual risk behaviors (Olley et al. 2017).

Slavin et al. (2017) examined links between lifetime cannabis use and hypersexuality among 228 university students. They conducted a hierarchical regression adjusting for self-identified gender and alcohol use to evaluate the degree to which cannabis use and expectancies accounted for variance in hypersexuality. Cannabis use and hypersexuality were significantly and positively related, and after adjusting for covariates, cannabis perceptual and cognitive enhancement expectancies positively correlated with hypersexuality, whereas tension reduction and relaxation expectancies negatively correlated with hypersexuality. These authors further posited that future research should explore the prospective relationship between hypersexuality and positively and negatively reinforcing cannabis expectancies among cannabis users. Given the growing legislation of cannabis across the United States, more research is needed to examine the relationship between problematic cannabis use and CSB, particularly if sexual behaviors are paired with substance use.

Special Populations

Substance abuse/misuse and CSB have been explored in other populations. Among 1,214 men who have sex with men (Grov et al. 2010), researchers found frequent club drug use in the past 90 days (17.1%). Additionally, 30.5% of the sample received a positive score on a measure of sexual compulsivity (Kalichman and Rompa 1995). Sexual compulsivity was associated with HIV risk behaviors (e.g., unprotected anal sex, group sex), and men who had engaged in sex while under the influence of at least one of these drugs scored significantly higher on sexual compulsivity compared with men who had not (Grov et al. 2010).

Other studies have found similar relationships between CSB and HIV risk behaviors among men who have sex with men. Among 699 homosexual and bisexual men, researchers examined associations between sexual compulsivity, depression, child sexual abuse, and HIV risk. They found that men who engaged in high-risk sexual intercourse had 2.25 higher odds of reporting symptoms of sexual compulsivity. Moreover, they noted that sexual compulsivity was positively associated with being HIV positive and reporting unprotected anal intercourse, which is consistent with previous research (Parsons et al. 2012). Recently, Chumakov et al. (2019) examined CSB in a sample of HIV-infected men in a community-based sample in Russia. Results revealed that nearly one-third (29.5%) of the 119 men with HIV met criteria for CSBD. Furthermore, CSB in men who have sex with men was positively associated with a history of illicit drug use, stimulant use, and alcohol abuse. Researchers concluded that CSB could be a significant risk factor for HIV infection among vulnerable groups. However, the relationship between stimulant use (e.g., methamphetamine, cocaine) and CSB requires further study among clinical and nonclinical populations.

Another population considered at risk for CSB is U.S. military veterans. Among 820 post-9/11 U.S. military veterans, Kraus et al. (2017) found that more men (13.8%) than women (4.3%) endorsed CSB-related symptoms. After adjusting for significant sociodemographics, results indicated that gambling, suicidality, and sexually transmitted infections were significantly associated with male CSB. No significant differences were noted between men with or without CSB-related symptoms for alcohol use disorder (30.9% vs. 20.2%) or drug dependence (5.9% vs. 5.9%). A recent study by Moisson et al. (2019) examined psychopathology and hypersexuality in 283 post-9/11 U.S. military veterans and found that 39.1% of the sample met lifetime criteria for alcohol use disorder. A history of alcohol use disorder was positively associated with problematic pornography use and hypersexuality. Such findings suggest that further screening for SUDs and hypersexuality among U.S. veterans is strongly warranted.

TREATMENT RECOMMENDATIONS

Few treatment studies involving placebo control groups, randomization, and considerable sample sizes have been conducted. A number of psychotherapies have been developed and piloted for CSBs, including the problematic use of pornography. Preliminary evidence suggests that cognitive-behavioral therapy (Hallberg et al. 2017), ACT (Crosby and Twohig 2016), and mindfulness-based approaches (Brem et al. 2017b; Reid et al. 2014) may be helpful. Given the similarities between SUDs and CSBD, adapting efficacious treatments for SUDs for individuals with CSB may be an efficient way to develop treatments (Kraus et al. 2016). Although some treatments (mindfulness-based approaches, ACT) appear helpful when treating patients with CSB, further work is needed to develop and test the efficacy of treatments that target both CSB and substance use. Given that many people who report issues with CSB also experience intense feelings of shame and guilt (Gilliland et al. 2011), we posit that the use of mindfulness-based approaches (including ACT) may be suitable to address both internal negative feelings and cognitions commonly found in those seeking treatment. Moreover, treatment approaches that provide patients with a greater focus on awareness of interoceptive processes through mind/body connectedness should also be explored (Blycker and Potenza 2018).

One possible treatment worth exploring with clients could be mindfulness-based relapse prevention (MBRP) (Bowen et al. 2009). MBRP teaches participants to recognize early warning signs of relapse and increases awareness of internal (i.e., emotional and cognitive) and external (i.e., situational) cues associated with prior substance use. Participants develop effective coping skills, enhance self-efficacy while also learning basic skills to raise awareness of triggers, monitor internal reactions, and foster more skillful behavioral choices. MBRP focuses on increasing acceptance and tolerance of positive and negative physical, emotional, and cognitive states (e.g., cravings) by decreasing the perceived need to alleviate associated discomfort by engaging in substance use (Bowen et al. 2009). As discussed elsewhere, overlapping features exist between CSB and SUDs (Kraus et al. 2016). Specifically, evidence suggests that CSB is associated with altered functioning in brain regions and networks implicated in sensitization, habituation, impulse dyscontrol, and reward processing in patterns such as substance, gambling, and gaming addictions (Kowalewska et al. 2018). Therefore, we think treatments such as mindfulness, ACT, or MBRP would have maximum benefits in treating multiple issues while enhancing treatment outcomes for patients with CSB and co-occurring substance use issues because they target some of the same proposed neurobiological pathways in the brain.

CASE EXAMPLES

Mr. C

Mr. C was a U.S. Army veteran, a cisgender heterosexual male who was estranged from his wife. He was in his mid-50s and presented for treatment of problematic pornography and cocaine use. Mr. C's CSBs first involved the use of crack cocaine, having casual sex with women (often prostitutes), and paying them with drugs. Mr. C would engage in these risky behaviors and then experience extreme fear of acquiring a sexually transmitted disease. He described an inability to refrain from engaging in paid sex, coupled with long periods of cocaine use (i.e., binges lasting 2–3 days). Mr. C engaged in paid sex and cocaine use for about 1 year before he was introduced to the idea of using pornography and cocaine together. Subsequently, he would go through periods in which he would exclusively use pornography. He reported intense urges to view pornography, coupled with frequent/repeated masturbation, and failed attempts to moderate or quit using pornography and to limit his exposure to it via his cellphone. He would engage in extended viewing of pornography (several hours or longer) when his urges became intense. Within 3 days, on average, he would experience an intense craving for cocaine and would begin to use again, coupled with pornography use.

Mr. C married his now-estranged wife after his year of crack cocaine use and casual sex. His use of pornography significantly impaired their marriage and ultimately contributed to their separation. He reported failed attempts at maintaining employment because of the long periods of binges (cocaine and pornography) that would consume him for days on end. He described his pornography and cocaine use as "compulsive": he denied experiencing intense feelings of pleasure from pornography, but was unable to cope with his intense urges and emotional states. Pornography use (followed by cocaine use) was his primary coping strategy for stress and negative moods.

In Mr. C's first session, he was cautious about what he shared, and in the initial stages of treatment he only felt comfortable discussing his substance abuse. After becoming more comfortable in treatment, he began to identify the pornography use as a primary concern; however, he was not consistent in attending scheduled individual sessions. Mr. C was also referred to group psychotherapy. He successfully attended four sessions and thought that the skills he learned were helpful in managing his urges to use pornography.

Mr. C had been raised in an urban area where he was exposed to considerable violence and reported being both a victim and a perpetrator. Additionally, he described a history of childhood sexual abuse; however, he was reluctant to describe the details of this traumatic experience. He reported joining the army at age 18 with the hope of escaping the chaos of his childhood environment. As he discussed in therapy, Mr. C used pornography as a way of coping with his isolation and low-esteem, and viewing pornography served as a way for him to self-soothe and escape the loneliness he felt. The therapist communicated to Mr. C the view that he was hardworking, intelligent, pleasant, gentle, likable, and adaptive. This last characteristic was demonstrated by the reduction in pornography viewing he had achieved through behavioral treatments that targeted his sexual urges (and thoughts) and provided greater insight into the motivations for use and the impacts of his behaviors. This led to a harm reduction approach involving casual sex versus problematic pornography use. Mr. C reported sustained abstinence from cocaine use over the course of treatment.

Mr. F

Mr. F was a Catholic, widowed, Vietnam-era U.S. military veteran in his late 60s. He presented with a history of paying for sex with other individuals. Mr. F had a long history of psychosis, beginning at age 15, which resulted in a psychiatric hospitalization. He had been diagnosed with undifferentiated schizophrenia in his 20s. An episode of psychosis occurred when he was in the military, and at that time he was given a medical discharge.

Mr. F unexpectedly lost his wife approximately 8 years ago, which was the precipitating factor for his CSB. He enrolled in a phone service by which he would be connected with women for the purpose of a date and paid sex. In addition, he would attend a specific strip club where he would pay for sexual services. Mr. F reported that he would attend the strip club earlier in the day so that he could "hang out" with the women before their performances.

Mr. F sought therapy for CSB and met with a doctoral-level psychology intern for approximately 10 sessions. Mr. F and his therapist worked on processing the shame he felt around paying others for sex, because many of these individuals would then use the money for drug use. Through therapy, Mr. F also able to share for the first time that he had also had sexual encounters with men. These encounters led him to question his sexual identity, and this was a focus of treatment. Specifically, Mr. F was provided with psychoeducation and validation related to sexual *behaviors* versus sexual *identity*. Mr. F was already connected with the Veterans Administration hospital (where the clinic was located) and engaged in various services throughout the hospital; this connection helped keep him out of the inpatient hospital for nearly 10 years despite his serious mental illness. Moreover, this current engagement in non-CSB mental health services supported his overall recovery and stability.

GAPS IN THE LITERATURE AND FUTURE DIRECTIONS

Currently, there are multiple gaps in understanding regarding CSBs, as detailed elsewhere (Grubbs et al. 2020; Kraus et al. 2016). Most research has focused on white heterosexual males, and more research is needed in other populations, particularly among individuals with co-occurring substance use. With the inclusion of CSBD in ICD-11, more research is needed to investigate multiple aspects (Kraus et al. 2018) as we determine the diagnostic criteria that describe CSB. Data are limited on the prevalence and manifestation of CSBs in various groups, including older adults and those with medical or psychiatric illnesses. CSBs may present in different ways in these groups compared with other groups. More work is also needed among LGBTQ individuals who have been understudied in the literature, except for homosexual or bisexual men who have sex with men, and the emphasis has been focused on HIV-risk behaviors (Yoon et al. 2016). Growing evidence suggests that the initiation of methamphetamine use may increase sexual risk behavior among HIV-uninfected men who have sex with men (Hoenigl et al. 2016). Research is still evolving on whether stimulants (e.g., methamphetamine, cocaine) are merely associated with high-risk behavior or if stimulant use leads to high-risk behaviors such as unprotected vaginal or anal sex, frequent casual sex behaviors, or compulsive masturbation. Given that much of what we know about CSB and substance use is drawn from cross-sectional data, we cannot speak to causation. Studies using a longitudinal panel design examining CSB over the lifespan that include measures of psychopathology, psychosocial functioning, substance use, sexual behaviors, and other important factors could help identify both risk and protective factors for CSB across diverse groups (e.g., those who self-identify as women, persons of color) (see Kowalewska et al. 2020 for discussion).

Additional research is needed to study the efficacy of treatments (e.g., cognitive-behavioral therapy, ACT, pharmacotherapy) for individuals with CSB and substance use (Gola and Potenza 2016; Kraus et al. 2015). We suspect that treatments targeting the mechanisms of craving and compulsions that overlap with SUDs would be helpful for further study. CSBD has recently been included in ICD-11, which represents a significant step forward in providing care for people with this diagnosis. Moving forward, more research is needed into types of CSBs, the defining characteristics of individuals with forms of CSBD, and the development of empirically validated policies and prevention and treatment approaches to promote individual and public health.

REFERENCES

American Psychiatric Association: Diagnostic and Statistical Manual of Mental Disorders, 5th Edition. Arlington, VA, American Psychiatric Association, 2013

Black DW, Kehrberg LL, Flumerfelt DL, Schlosser SS: Characteristics of 36 subjects reporting compulsive sexual behavior. Am J Psychiatry 154:243–249, 1997

Blycker GR, Potenza MN: A mindful model of sexual health: a review and implications of the model for the treatment of individuals with compulsive sexual behavior disorder. J Behav Addict 7:917–929, 2018

Bowen S, Chawla N, Collins SE, et al: Mindfulness-based relapse prevention for substance use disorders: a pilot efficacy trial. Subst Abuse 30:295–305, 2009

Brem MJ, Shorey RC, Anderson S, Stuart GL: Depression, anxiety, and compulsive sexual behaviour among men in residential treatment for substance use disorders: the role of experiential avoidance. Clin Psychol Psychother 24, 1246–1253, 2017a

Brem MJ, Shorey RC, Anderson S, Stuart GL: Dispositional mindfulness, shame, and compulsive sexual behaviors among men in residential treatment for substance use disorders. Mindfulness 8:1552–1558, 2017b

Brem MJ, Shorey RC, Anderson S, Stuart GL: Does experiential avoidance explain the relationships between shame, PTSD symptoms, and compulsive sexual behaviour among women in substance use treatment? Clin Psychol Psychother 25(5):692–700, 2018

Bryan AD, Schmiege SJ, Magnan RE: Marijuana use and risky sexual behavior among high-risk adolescents: trajectories, risk factors, and event-level relationships. Dev Psychol 48(5):1429, 2012

Carnes P, Murray RE, Charpentier L: Bargains with chaos: Sex addicts and addiction interaction disorder. Sexual Addiction and Compulsivity 12(2–3):79–120, 2005

Carnes P, Green B, Carnes S: The same yet different: refocusing the Sexual Addiction Screening Test (SAST) to reflect orientation and gender. Sexual Addiction and Compulsivity 17(1):7–30, 2010

Carvalho J, Guerra L, Neves S, Nobre PJ: Psychopathological predictors characterizing sexual compulsivity in a nonclinical sample of women. J Sex Marital Ther 41:467–480, 2015

Chumakov EM, Petrova NN, Kraus SW: Compulsive sexual behavior in HIV-infected men in a community based sample, Russia. Sexual Addiction and Compulsivity 26(1–2):164–175, 2019

Crosby JM, Twohig MP: Acceptance and commitment therapy for problematic internet pornography use: a randomized trial. Behav Ther 47:355–366, 2016

Dembo R, Briones-Robinson R, Barrett K, et al: Brief intervention for truant youth sexual risk behavior and marijuana use. J Child Adolesc Subst Abuse 23(5):318–333, 2014

Deneke E, Knepper C, Green BA, Carnes PJ: Comparative study of three levels of care in a substance use disorder inpatient facility on risk for sexual addiction. Sexual Addiction and Compulsivity 22(2):109–125, 2015

Dickenson JA, Gleason N, Coleman E, Miner MH: Prevalence of distress associated with difficulty controlling sexual urges, feelings, and behaviors in the United States. JAMA Network Open 1(7):e184468, 2018

Diehl A, Clemente J, Pillon SC, et al: Early childhood maltreatment experience and later sexual behavior in Brazilian adults undergoing treatment for substance dependence. Braz J Psychiatry 41(3):199–207, 2019

Elmquist J, Shorey RC, Anderson S, Stuart GL: The relation between compulsive sexual behaviors and aggression in a substance-dependent population. J Aggress Maltreat Trauma 25(1)110–124, 2016

Erez G, Pilver CE, Potenza MN: Gender-related differences in the associations between sexual impulsivity and psychiatric disorders. J Psychiatr Res 55:117–125, 2014

Farré JM, Fernandez-Aranda F, Granero R, et al: Sex addiction and gambling disorder: similarities and differences. Compr Psychiatry 56:59–68, 2015

Gilliland R, South M, Carpenter BN, Hardy SA: The roles of shame and guilt in hypersexual behavior. Sexual Addiction and Compulsivity 18:12–29, 2011

Gola M, Potenza MN: Paroxetine treatment of problematic pornography use: a case series. J Behav Addict 5:529–532, 2016

Gola M, Potenza MN: The proof of the pudding is in the tasting: data are needed to test models and hypotheses related to compulsive sexual behaviors. Arch Sex Behav 47(5):1323–1325, 2018

Grov C, Parsons JT, Bimbi DS: Sexual compulsivity and sexual risk in gay and bisexual men. Arch Sex Behav 39(4):940–949, 2010

Grubbs JB, Grant JT, Lee BN, et al: Sexual addiction 25 years on: a systematic and methodological review of empirical literature and an agenda for future research. Clin Psychol Rev 82:101925, 2020

Hallberg J, Kaldo V, Arver S, et al: A cognitive-behavioral therapy group intervention for hypersexual disorder: a feasibility study. J Sex Med 14(7):950–958, 2017

Hoenigl M, Chaillon A, Moore DJ, et al: Clear links between starting methamphetamine and increasing sexual risk behavior: a cohort study among men who have sex with men. J Acquir Immune Defic Syndr 71(5):551–557, 2016

Kafka MP: Hypersexual disorder: a proposed diagnosis for DSM-V. Arch Sex Behav 39(2):377–400, 2010

Kafka MP, Hennen J: A DSM-IV Axis I comorbidity study of males (N=120) with paraphilias and paraphilia-related disorders. Sex Abuse 14(4):349–366, 2002

Kalichman SC, Rompa D: Sexual sensation seeking and sexual compulsivity scales: reliability, validity, and predicting HIV risk behavior. J Pers Assess 65(3):586–601, 1995

Kowalewska E, Grubbs JB, Potenza MN, et al: Neurocognitive mechanisms in compulsive sexual behavior disorder. Curr Sex Health Rep 10:255–264, 2018

Kowalewska E, Gola M, Kraus SW, Lew-Starowicz M: Spotlight on compulsive sexual behavior disorder: a systematic review of research on women. Neuropsychiatr Dis Treat 16:2025–2043, 2020

Kraus SW, Meshberg-Cohen S, Martino S, et al: Treatment of compulsive pornography use with naltrexone: a case report. Am J Psychiatry 172:1260–1261, 2015

Kraus SW, Voon V, Potenza MN: Should compulsive sexual behavior be considered an addiction? Addiction 111(12):2097–2106, 2016

Kraus SW, Martino S, Potenza MN, et al: Examining compulsive sexual behavior and psychopathology among a sample of postdeployment U.S. male and female military veterans. Mil Psychol 29:143–156, 2017

Kraus SW, Krueger RB, Briken P, et al: Compulsive sexual behaviour disorder in the ICD-11. World Psychiatry 17(1):109–110, 2018

Kuzma JM, Black DW: Epidemiology, prevalence, and natural history of compulsive sexual behavior. Psychiatr Clin North Am 31:603–611, 2008

Moisson J, Potenza MN, Shirk SD, et al: Psychopathology and hypersexuality among veterans with and without histories of alcohol-use disorders. Am J Addict 28:398–404, 2019

Odlaug BL, Lust K, Schreiber LR, et al: Compulsive sexual behavior in young adults. Ann Clin Psychiatry 25:193–200, 2013

Olley BO, Oladele O, Adekeye OA: Does depression mediate the effect of sexual compulsivity in sexual risk behavior among cannabis users in Nigeria?, in Perspective on Drugs, Alcohol and Society in Africa, Vol 4. Abuja, CRISA, 2017, pp 37–42

Parsons JT, Grov C, Golub SA: Sexual compulsivity, co-occurring psychosocial health problems, and HIV risk among gay and bisexual men: further evidence of a syndemic. Am J Public Health 102:156–162, 2012

Raymond NC, Coleman E, Miner MH: Psychiatric comorbidity and compulsive/impulsive traits in compulsive sexual behavior. Compr Psychiatry 44:370–380, 2003

Reid RC, Bramen JE, Anderson A, Cohen MS: Mindfulness, emotional dysregulation, impulsivity, and stress proneness among hypersexual patients. J Clin Psychol 70:313–321, 2014

Scanavino MdT, Ventuneac A, Abdo CHN, et al: Compulsive sexual behavior and psychopathology among treatment-seeking men in São Paulo, Brazil. Psychiatry Res 209(3):518–524, 2013

Shorey RC, Elmquist J, Gawrysiak MJ, et al: The relationship between mindfulness and compulsive sexual behavior in a sample of men in treatment for substance use disorders. Mindfulness 7:866–873, 2016

Slavin MN, Kraus SW, Ecker A, et al: Marijuana use, marijuana expectancies, and hypersexuality among college students. Sexual Addiction and Compulsivity 24(4):248–256, 2017

Stavro K, Rizkallah E, Dinh-Williams L, et al: Hypersexuality among a substance use disorder population. Sexual Addiction and Compulsivity 20(3):210–216, 2013

Štulhofer A, Jurin T, Briken P: Is high sexual desire a facet of male hypersexuality? Results from an online study. J Sex Marital Ther 42:665–680, 2016

World Health Organization: International Classification of Diseases and Related Health Problems, 11th Revision. Geneva, World Health Organization, 2019

Yoon IS, Houang ST, Hirshfield S, Downing MJ: Compulsive sexual behavior and HIV/STI risk: a review of current literature. Curr Addict Rep 3(4):387–399, 2016

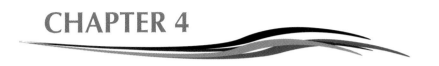

CHAPTER 4

The Internet and CSBD

Cristina Giménez-García, Ph.D.
Rafael Ballester-Arnal, Ph.D.
Kristian Daneback, Ph.D.

The term *online sexual activities* (OSA) refers to a range of online activities that are sexual in nature. However, no definition has been agreed upon, so making comparisons between studies has been difficult. It has been suggested that OSA may be broken down into six areas of sexuality (Döring 2009), as illustrated in Table 4–1. This division into categories is meaningful not only because of the different character of each of these areas but also because the categories are often associated with distinct types of internet services (e.g., websites, social networking sites, online content platforms).

Research literature has documented the use of the internet for sexual purposes for more than 20 years. In the mid-1990s, these publications were based on case studies and clinical reports as well as other, more speculative narratives on the possible benefits and risks of internet sexuality. As more empirical data were collected, including large-scale survey studies around the time of the new millennium, researchers began to

Table 4–1.   Description of online sexual activities and related areas
of sexuality

Online sexual activities	Areas of sexuality
Searching for information about sexual response, dysfunctions, HIV prevention	Sex education: information and knowledge
Viewing pornography or explicit sexual content.	Sexual desire, fantasies, and stimulation
Making sexual contacts	Sexual and affective interaction: experience with steady or casual partners
Sexual identity–based subcultures	Sexual identity and orientation in a nonheteronormative context
Sex products	Sexual stimulation and behaviors
Sex work	Sexual interaction: financial transactions

map out user demographics and usage patterns and conduct more advanced multivariate analyses. As a result, today we have a more empirically informed and detailed body of knowledge on which to theorize
about the future.

However, there are problems with self-selected samples as well as
the broad variety of OSA. We do not know the prevalence of engagement
in OSA in the general population; for example, a four-country (Canada,
Germany, Sweden, and the United States) comparison of young people
revealed that 30.8% had engaged in cybersex and 76.5% had accessed
sexually stimulating material (Döring et al. 2015). Regarding user profiles, a two-country comparison revealed that around 71% of Spanish
and 86% of Mexican young people between 15 and 18 years old reported
recreational use of "internet sex" (Ballester-Arnal et al. 2017). At the
same time, around 29% and 14% of these respondents, respectively, reported some type of interference, such as low self-control to avoid internet sex or spending more money than planned.

Reports concerning the outcomes of OSA have pointed in different di-
rections. Some studies suggest negative as well as both neutral and positive outcomes for individuals—even from engaging in the same OSA.
However, although it seems as though engaging in OSA is not problematic for most people—and even beneficial for some—empirical evidence
suggests that, for some people, OSA may interfere with their everyday
lives. Online sexual problems manifest in different ways and are related
to specific activities. The problems may involve compulsivity, be finan-

cial, or result in personal negative consequences on- or offline. Prior research suggests that online sexual problems are more common among males than females and among bisexuals and homosexuals in particular; however, for these latter populations, engagement in OSA may actually be more positive than for heterosexual users.

This chapter focuses on when engagement in OSA may result in online sexual problems, particularly internet compulsive sexual behavior disorder (CSBD) and proposals for treatment.

THE INTERNET AND COMPULSIVE SEXUAL BEHAVIOR: UNDERLYING FACTORS

OSA may promote sexual development based on new knowledge, having access to open-minded attitudes and people with similar interests, or discovering various sexual experiences (Döring et al. 2015). However, at the same time, internet sex might interfere in psychological well-being, particularly when CSBD is present (Cooper et al. 2000). In line with ICD-11 (World Health Organization 2019) in particular, CSBD is characterized by persistent problems controlling sexual impulses or urges to engage in sex over an extended period of time (e.g., ≥6 months) that interfere with important areas in daily life and causing distress.

Mr. D

Mr. D was a 37-year-old male who had been married for 6 years. He searched for pornography on the internet and participated in online sexual chats to reduce discomfort and to calm the sexual excitement that preceded his urge to go online. Chatting and using pornography usually reduced his anxiety and sadness and, most of the time, helped him feel more desirable, and balanced his self-esteem. He masturbated regularly while viewing pornography and chatting, about 10 times per week, and these primarily provided his preferred sexual stimulation. In the beginning, 3 years earlier, he believed that he could control his OSA ("I only use internet sex sporadically") and feelings of guilt were nonexistent ("Cybersex doesn't cause any harm"). He remembered that around the age of 16 he started to search for pornography on the internet to assist with masturbation. Recently he recognized a need to increase the variety of sexual activities he engaged in as well as the time he spent online. Consequently, he expened around 20 hours per week for sexual satisfaction.

A few months earlier, Mr. D began to spend money in sex chatrooms. When he was online, the internet absorbed him, and his problems disappeared. However, sometimes, when he finished his OSA and realized the resulting negative consequences, he felt regret ("Oh, this is terrible. I can't arrive on time to my workshop. I really should give up cybersex. This will disrupt my life"). Most of the time, this ambivalence disappeared, and sexual thoughts and fantasies about his next online experience would suddenly appear in his mind until he engaged in cybersex again. Cybersex did not always satisfy him, and 6 months ago he tried to give it up, but he was only able to do so for 3 weeks. He returned to disregarding responsibilities, such as attending family meetings, finishing work tasks on time, or participating in certain workshops. The week before, his wife had become aware of his "second life"; she had woken up during the night and caught him by surprise. At that moment, she gave him an ultimatum: she would forgive his indiscretions once but not twice. For this main reason, Mr. D decided to seek help.

This case illustrates the main characteristics to cover criteria for CSBD suggested by the ICD-11, as well as scientific literature (Wéry and Billieux 2016).

First, Mr. D had lost control of his OSA, which he continued despite hurting other people and himself (Carnes 2000; Grov et al. 2008). Therefore, involvement in OSA seemed to be the most important motivation in his life. Even though he did not always obtain satisfaction from these activities (i.e., viewing pornography and participating in sexual chats), he repeated them nonetheless. In some cases, OSA takes up between 35 and 45 hours per week, extending the use of internet sex to other settings such as the workplace (Cooper et al. 2000, 2002). Most patients report disruptive and intrusive thoughts about internet sex similar to an obsessive disorder (Wéry and Billieux 2015), such as anticipating their connection, fantasizing about OSA, or deciding how hide their OSA from others. This may be related to thinking of desires and particularly associated with verbal perseveration (Allen et al. 2017). Moreover, Mr. D showed an ineffective emotional self-regulation, using internet sex to deal with his emotional discomfort (Carnes 1991; Goodman 1998). He illustrated a process in which his compulsive sexual behavior (CSB) online arose with the convergence of sexual thoughts, sexual arousal, and risk routines that promoted the accessibility of cybersex behaviors, although they later caused feelings of guilt and despair (Carnes et al. 2007).

These types of feelings related to guilt or shame are not sufficient in and of themselves to indicate a disorder. As Mr. D described, compulsive OSA could be linked to dissociation based on depersonalization and absorption when people are online (Chaney and Burns-Wortham 2014). A wide variety of practices are possible, from viewing pornography to practicing cybersex via webcams. Most of the time, patients seek help from professionals when they recognize the impact that their CSB has had on their life or, as in the case of Mr. D, when someone sets an ultimatum (Griffiths 2012). The patient may have engaged in CSB for many years, ignoring the negative consequences. In any case, the perceived CSBD and resulting distress may be related to moral values apart from the seriousness of the diagnoses (Grubbs et al. 2018). In addition to compulsive OSA, some patients show other comorbid problems, such as depression or anxiety disorders (Stein et al. 2001).

WHO IS MORE LIKELY TO EXPERIENCE COMPULSIVE ONLINE SEXUAL BEHAVIOR?

In order to specify risky profiles, the literature provides possible reasons why some people are more likely than others to develop CSBD related to internet sexual activity. Although online CSB can occur irrespective of sex, ethnicity, or sexual orientation (Green et al. 2012), different personal traits and sociodemographic characteristics may be associated with risk. The internet itself presents some characteristics that may also facilitate CSBD. Cybersex is possible through easy accessibility, perceived anonymity, and affordability, as identified by Cooper (1998) in his "Triple A Engine" model as well as additional traits provided by Carnes et al. (2007) in their Cyberhex model. The internet would be "imposing," taking into account that in everyday life its use is almost mandatory in our society. The internet is both isolating and interactive because it allows people to search for sexual material away from others, in private, but facilitates connections with other people, providing a sense of belonging to a community (Döring 2009). Therefore, it provides a variety of uses, from isolated activities (e.g., viewing cyberpornography or searching for sexual information) to social activities (e.g., interacting with other users, participating in sexual chats or sexual meetings via webcam), including the possibility of moving to offline interactions. In this context, people who use internet sex to increase or improve their sexual pleasure and desire (e.g., watching pornography or engaging in sex via webcam) are more likely to report problematic use than are those who use the internet to improve their knowledge (Cooper et al. 2001). In addition, the literature has reported other consequences, such as exposure to HIV among those who have sex with partners they meet online (Siegel et al. 2017).

Regarding social and demographic variables, males seem more likely to report online CSB than females (Ballester-Arnal et al. 2014; Daneback et al. 2006; Giordano and Cashwell 2017). However, the literature reports fewer differences between males and females when some variables, such as sexual functioning problems or trait sexual motivation, mediate its use (Blais-Lecours et al. 2016; Stark et al. 2017). In addition, as suggested by Kafka (2010), most of those diagnosed with CSBD are older than 18, although some cases have been reported among adolescents as well (Ballester 2006). Past research has also pointed to higher-level education as a risk factor (Ross et al. 2012).

Concerning psychological profiles, the literature reveals various underlying factors. For example, users' motives for engaging in OSA are relevant factors in problematic cybersex behavior (Castro-Calvo et al. 2018b). Thus, people who use OSA to cope with dissatisfaction, regulate their mood, and avoid loneliness are more likely to experience problematic usage (Reid et al. 2011; Wéry and Billieux 2016). Moreover, driven by the internet's anonymity, fantasizing and being sexually active online for a long time has been related to problematic use (Reid et al. 2011; Stark et al. 2017; Wéry and Billieux 2016). In this sense, pleasure-seeking motives (Brown et al. 2017) and exploration of sexual fantasies could also be risk factors for developing online CSB (Cooper et al. 2001). Expecting arousal from cybersex would also have an impact, meaning that males and females who expect sexual pleasure and satisfaction from internet sex seem to be more likely to experience online CSB (Brand et al. 2011; Laier et al. 2014; Young 2008). As well as expectancies, other traits such as sexual sensation seeking and sexual compulsivity, as defined by Kalichman and Rompa (1995), have been related to predisposition to CSBD regardless of sexual orientation (Cooper et al. 2000; Laier et al. 2015). In this sense, people who report difficulty controlling sexual feelings, urges, and behaviors would reveal a greater tendency toward problematic use (Antons and Brand 2018; Laier and Brand 2014). In addition, as Sirianni and Vishwanath (2015) stated, people who report deficits of general self-regulation abilities would be more likely at risk for compulsive use of pornography.

Moreover, sexual dysfunctions such as erectile dysfunction or lower sexual satisfaction are related to compulsive OSA (Blais-Lecours et al. 2016; Voon et al. 2014). In this context, cybersex—particularly cyberpornography—may facilitate unadjusted expectations regarding sexual response and more concerns and less perceived self-control regarding sexuality that would decrease sexual satisfaction and functioning (Strasburger et al. 2012). In addition, OSA may maintain the sexual dysfunction when patients use it to obtain some type of sexual gratification while minimizing the disturbance of sexual dysfunction and avoiding their discomfort of coping with the problem. However, as Laier et al. (2015) stated, problematic use of the internet for sexual activities may not always be related to one's offline sexual behavior and experiences.

The literature suggests that being socialized in a conservative sexual culture (Ballester-Arnal et al. 2017; Earle and Earle 1995) and experiencing psychosocial trauma (Carnes 1993; Whitfield 1998) or sexual abuse (Schwartz and Southern 2000) may be related to online sexual problems.

However, the link with sexual abuse has been disputed (Chaney and Burns-Wortham 2014). Some studies have established a link between problematic use of internet sex and other psychopathological conditions (Laier et al. 2014), such as substance abuse (Wéry and Billieux 2015). In particular, positive attitudes about the consumption as well as the misuse of recreational drugs may hamper learning adjusted emotional regulation skills and may be associated with compulsive OSA (Castro-Calvo et al. 2016b). In addition, people with anxiety disorders (Santos et al. 2017), obsessive-compulsive symptoms, or feelings of loneliness (Young 2008) are more likely to experience problematic usage.

Therefore, a combination of evolutionary, biological, psychological, and social factors seems to increase the possibility of being at risk for online CSB (Poudat and Lagadec 2017), from the characteristics of the internet (e.g., accessibility, anonymity, and affordability) to the psychological profiles of the user (e.g., sexual sensation seeking, self-regulation abilities, or motivation of using the internet for sexual activities).

ASSESSMENT METHODS

Properly dealing with online CSB requires a thorough evaluation, in particular to determine whether the behavior is problematic and what underlying factors may play a role. To obtain a comprehensive perspective of a particular patient's profile, the therapist should explore the main problem as well as the related interference. In this context, semi-structured interviews that contain open questions and facilitate techniques such as listening reflectively or evaluating the patient's strengths could be effective (Ballester 2011). Besides the topography of actions and agreed-upon criteria (Carnes et al. 2007; Wéry and Billieux 2015; World Health Organization 2019), exploring the motivations, benefits, and interferences of the patient's maladaptive behavior is important for treatment. Moreover, evaluating the patient's ambivalence with motivational interviewing, accompanied by other proposals such as cognitive therapy, has proven to be effective (Del Giudice and Kutinsky 2007).

Because CSB is the result of a patient's experiences and background, LoPiccolo and Heiman (1978) suggested that some general aspects such as sexual development, environmental influences, or specific traumatic situations should be explored. Therefore, to comprehend what the patient's sexual problem is and why it persists, the therapist should initiate the interview by focusing on general aspects and subsequently move to questions of a more sexual nature. Regarding sexuality, exploring the patient's early psychosexual evolution (e.g., sex education, sexual debut, relationship experiences) is often worthwhile to evaluate potential underlying factors. In addition, the sexual assessment should contain an evaluation of present attitudes and behaviors (e.g., erotophilia/erotophobia, type of sexual practices, sexual orientation and desire, relationships) as well as the nature of the main sexual problem (e.g., topography, maintaining factors, disturbance, thoughts and feelings).

Patients who report CSB often face criticism from others and experience loneliness. Therapists should pay special attention to creating a friendly environment. In particular, the sexual component of this disorder usually increases the difficulty of detecting particular affected areas and symptoms in patients who are ashamed (Poudat and Lagadec 2017). Therapists should also review their own sexual values, concerns, and erotophilic attitudes to properly assess their clinical process and prevent unintentional discrimination (Jones and Tuttle 2012).

In addition to the clinical interview, some measures could improve the evaluation, such as the Sexual Addiction Screening Test–Revised (Carnes et al. 2010) and the Internet Sex Screening Test (Delmonico 1997) (Castro-Calvo et al. 2018a; Green et al. 2012). Grubbs et al. (2015) developed a short measure called the Cyber-Pornography Use Inventory–9 to assess compulsive pornography use via three subscales: Perceived Compulsivity, Access Efforts, and Emotional Distress. Moreover, a therapist would also need to assess specific modulating factors to design a comprehensive intervention (Ballester 2006). Some useful measures include the State-Trait Anxiety Inventory (Spielberger et al. 1970), the Beck Depression Inventory–II (Beck et al. 1996), the Sexual Sensation Seeking Scale and Sexual Compulsivity Scale (Kalichman and Rompa 1995), and the Rosenberg Self-Esteem Scale (Rosenberg 1965).

WHAT MAY WORK?

Although knowledge about CSBD, as well as some underlying factors, is increasing, not enough evidence yet supports a specific psychological or biological treatment (Kraus et al. 2016; Wéry and Billieux 2016). In fact, the great variability of profiles, ranging from paraphilic to sexual dysfunction comorbidity, as well as substance abuse or sexual-trauma consequences, increases its difficulty (Southern 2008).

Concerning biological treatment, some proposals such as serotonergic reuptake inhibitors (e.g., fluoxetine, sertraline, and citalopram) and opioid antagonists (e.g., naltrexone) might be effective to decrease some symptoms and behaviors. However, because there are significant gaps in past studies, not enough evidence is available to fully endorse them, and these results should therefore be treated with caution (Grant et al. 2013; Kraus et al. 2016).

Regarding psychological treatment, the literature has revealed some promising suggestions based on cognitive-behavioral therapy (Ballester 2006; Poudat and Lagadec 2017), readiness to change and motivational interviewing techniques (Orzack et al. 2006), 12-step programs (Delmonico et al. 2002), and acceptance and commitment therapy (Twohig and Crosby 2010). Most of these approaches last between 8 (Twohig and Crosby 2010) and 17 weekly sessions (Ballester 2006), revealing effectiveness in both group therapy (Orzack et al. 2006) and individual clinical interventions (Ballester 2006; Twohig and Crosby 2010). In terms of setting, most have been developed effectively for face-to-face interactions (Castro-Calvo and Ballester-Arnal 2013; Orzack et al. 2006), although other proposals support the potential effectiveness of online therapy based on its anonymity, accessibility, and confidentiality (Ballester 2011; Putnam 2000). This online context may be more accessible for patients with compulsivity who regularly search for information on the internet and could perceive it as a safer environment to escape social discrimination.

Taking account of patients' potential stigma, and based on available online facilities (Putnam 2000), some strategies such as online screening platforms would facilitate a first assessment as well as an introduction to patients (MacDonell and Prinz 2017). In this sense, online therapy may facilitate the anonymity and privacy of patients who participate from their home and provide more flexibility and accessibility regarding the time of day and the patient's (or therapist's) location. Some resources are readily available, such as the Adisex Project (https://adiccionalsexo.uji.es), which is aimed at Spanish-speaking people. After filling out the evaluation, patients receive feedback as well as an opportunity for therapy (Castro-Calvo et al. 2016a; Giménez-García et al. 2018).

Adjusting for effective treatment requires prioritizing the main objectives and components. For this purpose, therapy should contain a general objective that supports patients managing their urges to connect to the internet for sexual purposes and reinforcing their boundaries. Moreover, therapy should improve patients' skills and ability to modify maladaptive attitudes, thoughts, emotions, and behaviors in order to build a new pattern of sexual behaviors and life project if this is needed (Poudat and Lagadec 2017).

Despite the shortage of literature about treatment for CSBD, some clinical experiences may help therapists plan an effective psychological intervention (see Ballester 2006; Castro-Calvo and Ballester-Arnal 2013; Cooper et al. 2002; Orzack et al. 2006; Twohig and Crosby 2010). Following these, the treatment plan should include particular components such as a psychoeducational module, motivational interviewing, self-control

Table 4–2. Techniques for the specific compulsive sexual behavior disorder (CSBD) intervention

Situation	Technique	Example
Patients have problems understanding how factors facilitate their CSBD.	Analogy	Online sexual activities seem to decrease your depressed mood, as a pill would decrease physical pain.
Patients are not fully cognizant about interference and consequences.	Brainstorming based on open-ended question	What type of changes have you noticed since internet sex became more relevant in your life? Tell me all your thoughts without filtering them.
Patients have not recognized their problem as CSBD.	Case study	I will describe a case of CSBD. Do you recognize any characteristics or the situation as relevant to your situation?

training, exposure-response prevention, and a relapse-prevention module (Ballester 2015).

In general, there is agreement about the relevance of patients' understanding and acceptance of CSBD as well as their recognition of the harm caused by their problematic use of the internet for sexual purposes (Poudat and Lagadec 2017). Therefore, the first sessions should focus on psychoeducational efforts based on metaphors, descriptions, and quotidian comparisons to identify the main characteristics and agreed-upon criteria of CSBD, as well as the basic mechanisms that cause and maintain this problem (Table 4–2). In this context, describing the main modulators linked to the internet characteristics, the psychological and sexual profile of each patient, and their social environment would be relevant.

When patients analyze CSBD as a health problem in which different factors may have an influence, thus minimizing the social stigma, it is easier for them to normalize and accept their situation as a compulsive user of cybersex. For this purpose, the following information might be given to a patient who reports a significant moral burden related to social values, with the intention to remove the social weight of that patient's discomfort:

> The pattern of CSBD is very similar to other impulse-control disorders, such as kleptomania, and shares some characteristics such as a recurrent failure to control strong impulses to do something, for example, stealing objects. In this case, the mechanisms of reinforcement and maintenance are expressed in the sexual area, but beyond that, there are not many dif-

ferences in their bases. Therefore, this condition is just as legitimate as any other problem for which you might consult us. In any case, we will be working with the stigma or discomfort that some values may cause and why this happens.

As in other impulse-control disorders, a motivational component is required (Ballester 2015; Castro-Calvo and Ballester-Arnal 2013; Orzack et al. 2006; Twohig and Crosby 2010), especially when the patient reveals little concern about the problem. To obtain a global vision of a patient's problem, it is essential to initiate a process wherein the patient describes the benefits obtained and the problems caused by the cybersex behaviors. Moreover, to increase the patient's adjusted self-identification with the problem, reviewing some case studies in which patients realize coincidences may be useful. In cases in which a patient is hesitant to take measures to ameliorate the situation, emphasizing the patient's pain and discomfort about the CSBD over the primary rewards obtained from it could be effective. In any case, it would be important to include some details, for example, about the misconception of anonymity on the internet, thoughts that normalize the problem, and hazards related to CSBD, as well as some potential resources on how to deal with it. Moreover, some patients may report severe grief over losses related to ceasing their CSB (Carnes et al. 2007). The therapist should signify the meaning of cybersex, validate the emotional response, and evaluate how one could relocate new scenarios. In this phase, in line with Del Giudice and Kutinsky (2007), the therapist should tackle the patient's ambivalence about the OSA, reinforcing an internal locus of control and making visible the person's personal and social resources. Additional techniques such as behavioral contracts could facilitate better results (Canning 2002).

Considering the role of classic conditioning and associative learning in CSBD (Snagowski et al. 2016), many authors have supported the relevance of self-control training (Poudat and Lagadec 2017) that, as Carnes et al. (2007) stated, may include two related locations, external and internal boundaries. For this purpose, the functional analysis and its antecedent-behavior-consequence chart may increase the detailed knowledge about the internet sex episodes. Based on this information, environmental changes should be designed to facilitate online sexual abstention, such as searching for nonsexual information on the internet in public places (e.g., libraries or in therapy session), making some photos of relatives visible, or installing and using filtering software (Ballester 2006; Delmonico et al. 2002). This task requires a weekly check of each step as well as conceptualizing relapses as part of the process, which is in line with the transtheoretical model (Prochaska et al. 1992).

At the same time, when patients are trained in self-control techniques such as affect-regulation strategies, cognitive restructuring (i.e., cognitive therapy with common thoughts such as "Nobody loves me"; "If my wife realizes, she'll reject me"; or "I will not be able to overcome"), self-instruction, social skills, decision-making processes, reconditioning, relaxation, thought-stopping techniques, and healthy habits (Ballester 2006; Hagedorn and Juhnke 2005) and assimilated most of these techniques, exposure-response prevention exercises are developed. Consequently, the loss of control over consumption that facilitates the CSBD may be counteracted (Brand et al. 2011).

This stage may be one of the most complicated with this type of treatment; for this reason, including supportive techniques would improve effectiveness. For example, a contingency contract to reward each step would facilitate the goal, as would reinforcement of self-efficacy and internal locus of control to maintain self-expectations, for example, in a way similar to one used with an unconfident patient:

> You are working hard, and your progress is noticeable. I'm sure you will have more and more resources to control and regulate online sexual behavior. At this moment, experiencing certain sexual urges and a desire to connect is common. For this reason, we establish a period of environmental control that allows us to strengthen personal resources to deal with these situations more easily. Progress could seem to be hard, but step by step we can reinforce skills and possibilities of being successful.

In addition to these proposals, co-therapists such as partners, relatives, or friends would be convenient and potentially useful (Ballester 2015). Partners usually live in the same place and, most of the time, are close to the patient at the time and location where impulse control can be difficult and complicated. Acting as co-therapists also involves partners in the patients' treatment for a disorder that usually causes interference in the family and, particularly, in the patients themselves. Unfortunately, most patients keep their problem to themselves and deal with it in secret, making obtaining this type of social resource more difficult.

Treatment could also include an approach addressing comorbid situations, such as sexual dysfunction or gaps in sexual development, couples and relationship problems, loneliness, or past sexual aggression (Delmonico et al. 2002).

Finally, relapse prevention is an important component in the treatment of CSB (Castro-Calvo and Ballester-Arnal 2013). For this purpose, to avoid the possibility of abusing OSA and to promote healthier coping with risky situations (at least being able to stop cybersex and request support immediately), relapse-prevention measures would reinforce learning as well as self-efficacy. At this point, detecting triggers for the specific OSA and the underlying factors of relapses is essential. At the same time, identifying the most viable and effective mechanisms to avoid these triggers is also important. Moreover, adding an avoiding stimulus may be useful, such as patients writing an empathic personal letter to themselves that describes their understanding about urges, their motivations for avoiding cybersex, and strategies to not engage in it (Ballester 2006).

Although more evidence is needed to support a definitive protocol for treatment of online CSB, our understanding and experience allow us to suggest some relevant components and techniques that seem effective for patients while considering possible common traits related to other mental disorders and particular characteristics of CSBD (Ballester 2006; Castro-Calvo and Ballester-Arnal 2013; Orzack et al. 2006; Twohig and Crosby 2010). Future analyses should verify and study in depth the mechanisms of CSBD development, as well as what types of techniques allow effective treatment for patients. Future research should focus on what comes first—OSA or hypersexuality.

REFERENCES

Allen A, Kannis-Dymand L, Katsikitis M: Problematic internet pornography use: the role of craving, desire thinking, and metacognition. Addict Behav 70:65–71, 2017

Antons S, Brand M: Trait and state impulsivity in males with tendency towards internet-pornography-use disorder. Addict Behav 79:171–177, 2018

Ballester R: Psychological treatment for a cybersex addiction case, in Psychological Therapy for Children and Adolescents. Edited by Méndez F, Espada JP, Orgilés M. Madrid, Pirámide, 2006, pp 387–414

Ballester R: Cybersex addiction: nosology, prevalence and therapeutic approach. Presented at the V World Congress of Behavioural and Cognitive Therapies, Barcelona, Spain, July 11–14, 2011

Ballester R: Evaluation and treatment of cybersex addiction. Presented at IX Congreso de la Asociación Española de Psicología Clínica y Psicopatología, Valencia, Spain, October 23–24, 2015

Ballester-Arnal R, Castro-Calvo J, Gil-Llario MD, Giménez-García C: Relationship status as an influence on cybersex activity: cybersex, youth, and steady partner. J Sex Marital Ther 40:444–456, 2014

Ballester-Arnal R, Gil-Llario MD, Giménez-García C, et al: Sexuality in the internet era: expressions of Hispanic adolescent and young people. Sexual Addiction and Compulsivity 24(3):144–155, 2017

Beck AT, Steer RA, Brown GK: Manual for the Beck Depression Inventory–II. San Antonio, TX, Psychological Corporation, 1996

Blais-Lecours S, Vaillancourt-Morel MP, Sabourin S, Godbout N: Cyberpornography: time use, perceived addiction, sexual functioning, and sexual satisfaction. Cyberpsychol Behav Soc Netw 19(11):649–655, 2016

Brand M, Laier C, Pawlikowski M, et al: Watching pornographic pictures on the internet: role of sexual arousal ratings and psychological-psychiatric symptoms for using internet sex sites excessively. Cyberpsychol Behav Soc Netw 14(6):371–377, 2011

Brown CC, Durtschi JA, Carroll JS, Willoughby BJ: Understanding and predicting classes of college students who use pornography. Comput Human Behav 66:114–121, 2017

Canning M: Breaking through defenses, in Clinical Management of Sex Addiction. Edited by Carnes P, Adams K. New York, Brunner-Routledge, 2002, pp 31–44

Carnes P: Don't Call It Love: Recovery From Sexual Addiction. New York, Bantam Books, 1991

Carnes P: Addiction and post-traumatic stress: the convergence of victims' realities. Treating Abuse Today 3(13):5–11, 1993

Carnes P: Sexual addiction and compulsion: recognition, treatment, and recovery. CNS Spectr 5(10):63–72, 2000

Carnes P, Delmonico D, Griffin E, Moriarity J: In the Shadows of the Net: Breaking Free of Compulsive Online Sexual Behavior, 2nd Edition. Center City, MN, Hazelden, 2007

Carnes P, Green B, Carnes S: The same yet different: refocusing the Sexual Addiction Screening Test (SAST) to reflect orientation and gender. Sexual Addiction and Compulsivity 17(1):7–30, 2010

Castro-Calvo J, Ballester-Arnal R: Psychological evaluation and treatment for addictions: cocaine and cybersex, in Clinical Health Psychology. Edited by Ballester-Arnal R, Gil-Llario MD. Suffolk, UK, Pearson, 2013, pp 111–130

Castro-Calvo J, Ballester-Arnal R, Gil-Llario MD, Chica-Mingarro P: ADISEX: impact of a web for evaluating and treating cybersex addiction. Paper presented at the 18th Latin American Congress of Sexology and Sex Education. Madrid, Spain, September 28–October 1, 2016a

Castro-Calvo J, Ballester-Arnal R, Gil-Llario MD, et al: Common etiological pathways between toxic substance use, internet and cybersex addiction: the role of expectancies and antisocial deviance proneness. Comput Human Behav 63:383–391, 2016b

Castro-Calvo J, Ballester-Arnal R, Billieux J, et al: Spanish validation of the Sexual Addiction Screening Test. J Behav Addict 7(3):584–600, 2018a

Castro-Calvo J, Giménez-García C, Gil-Llario MD, Ballester-Arnal R: Motives to engage in online sexual activities and their links to excessive and problematic use: a systematic review. Curr Addict Rep 5:491–510, 2018b

Chaney M, Burns-Wortham C: The relationship between online sexual compulsivity, dissociation, and past child abuse among men who have sex with men. J LGBT Issues Couns 8:146–163, 2014

Cooper A: Sexuality and the internet: surfing into the new millennium. Cyberpsychology and Behavior 1(2):187–193, 1998

Cooper A, Delmonico D, Burg R: Cybersex users, abusers, and compulsives: new findings and implications. Sexual Addiction and Compulsivity 7(1):5–29, 2000

Cooper A, Griffin-Shelley E, Delmonico DL, Mathy RM: Online sexual problems: assessment and predictive variables. Sexual Addiction and Compulsivity 8(3–4):267–285, 2001

Cooper A, McLoughlin I, Reich P, Kent-Ferraro J: Virtual sexuality in the work-place: a wake-up call for clinicians, employers, and employees, in Sex and the Internet: A Guidebook for Clinicians. Edited by Cooper A. New York, Routledge, 2002, pp 109–128

Daneback K, Ross MW, Mansson SA: Characteristics and behaviors of sexual compulsives who use the internet for sexual purposes. Sexual Addiction and Compulsivity 13:53–67, 2006

Del Giudice MJ, Kutinsky J: Applying motivational interviewing to the treatment of sexual compulsivity and addiction. Sexual Addiction and Compulsivity 14(4):303–319, 2007

Delmonico DL: Internet Sex Screening Test, 1997. Available at: http://www.sexhelp.com. Accessed May 15, 2010.

Delmonico DL, Griffin E, Carnes PJ: Treating online compulsive sexual behavior: when cybersex is the drug of choice, in Sex and the Internet: A Guidebook for Clinicians. Edited by Cooper A. New York, Routledge, 2002, pp 147–167

Döring N: The internet's impact on sexuality: a critical review of 15 years of research. Comput Human Behav 25(5):1089–1101, 2009

Döring N, Daneback K, Shaughnessy K, et al: Online sexual activity experiences among college students: a four-country comparison. Arch Sex Behav 46(6):1641–1652, 2015

Earle RH, Earle MR: Sex Addiction: Case Studies and Management. New York, Brunner/Mazel, 1995

Giménez-García C, Castro-Calvo J, Ballester-Arnal R, et al: ADISEX: three-year experience evaluation and treating cybersex addition on the internet. Presented at XXVII Meeting of SPCV Psychiatry and New Technologies, Castelló, Spain, May 11–12, 2018

Giordano AL, Cashwell C: Cybersex addiction among college students: a prevalence study. Sexual Addiction and Compulsivity 24(1):1–11, 2017

Goodman A: Sexual addiction: the new frontier. The Counselor 16:17–26, 1998

Grant JE, Schreiber LRN, Odlaug BL: Phenomenology and treatment of behavioural addictions. Can J Psychiatry 58(5):252–259, 2013

Green BA, Carnes S, Carnes PJ, Weinman EA: Cybersex addiction patterns in a clinical sample of homosexual, heterosexual, and bisexual men and women. Sexual Addiction and Compulsivity 19:77–98, 2012

Griffiths MD: Internet sex addiction: a review of empirical research. Addiction Research and Theory 20(2):111–124, 2012

Grov C, Bamonte A, Fuentes A, et al: Exploring the internet's role in sexual compulsivity and out of control sexual thoughts/behaviour: a qualitative study of gay and bisexual men in New York City. Cult Health Sex 10(2):107–125, 2008

Grubbs JB, Volk F, Exline JJ, Pargament KI: IP use: perceived addiction, psychological distress, and the validation of a brief measure. J Sex Marital Ther 41:83–106, 2015

Grubbs JB, Wilt JA, Exline JJ, et al: Moral disapproval and perceived addiction to internet pornography: a longitudinal examination. Addiction 113(3):496–506, 2018

Hagedorn WB, Juhnke GA: Treating the sexually addicted patient: establishing a need for increased counselor awareness. Journal of Addictions and Offender Counseling 25:66–86, 2005

Jones KE, Tuttle AE: Clinical and ethical considerations for the treatment of cybersex addiction for marriage and family therapists. Journal of Couple and Relationship Therapy 11:274–290, 2012

Kafka MP: Hypersexual disorder: a proposed diagnosis for DSM-V. Arch Sex Behav 39(2):377–400, 2010

Kalichman SC, Rompa D: Sexual sensation seeking and sexual compulsivity scales: reliability, validity and predicting HIV risk behavior. J Pers Assess 65(3):586–601, 1995

Kraus SW, Voon V, Potenza MN: Should compulsive sexual behavior be considered an addiction? Addiction 111(12):2097–2106, 2016

Laier C, Brand M: Empirical evidence and theoretical considerations on factors contributing to cybersex addiction from a cognitive-behavioral view. Sexual Addiction and Compulsivity 21(4):305–321, 2014

Laier C, Pekal J, Brand M: Cybersex addiction in heterosexual female users of internet pornography can be explained by gratification hypothesis. Cyberpsychol Behav Soc Netw 17(8):575–580, 2014

Laier C, Pekal J, Brand M: Sexual excitability and dysfunctional coping determine cybersex addiction in homosexual males. Cyberpsychol Behav Soc Netw 18(10):575–580, 2015

LoPiccolo J, Heiman J: Sexual Assessment and History Interview, in Handbook of Sex Therapy. Edited by LoPiccolo J, LoPiccolo L. New York, Plenum, 1978, pp 103–112

MacDonell KW, Prinz RJ: A review of technology-based youth and family focused interventions. Clin Child Fam Psychol Rev 20(2):185–200, 2017

Orzack M, Volusse A, Wolf D, Hennen J: An ongoing study of group treatment for men involved in problematic Internet-enabled sexual behavior. Cyberpsychology and Behavior 9(3):348–360, 2006

Poudat F, Lagadec M: Cybersex addiction and cognitive behavioral therapy. Journal de Thérapie Comportementale et Cognitive 27(3):138–146, 2017

Prochaska J, DiClemente C, Norcross JC: In search of how people change: applications to addictive behaviors. Am Psychol 47(9):1102–1114, 1992

Putnam DE: Initiation and maintenance of online sexual compulsivity: implications for assessment and treatment. Cyberpsychology and Behavior 3(4):553–563, 2000

Reid RC, Li DS, Gilliland R, et al: Reliability, validity, and psychometric development of the Pornography Consumption Inventory in a sample of hypersexual men. J Sex Marit Ther 37(5):359–385, 2011

Rosenberg M: Society and the Adolescent Self-Image. Princeton, NJ, Princeton University Press, 1965

Ross MW, Månsson SA, Daneback K: Prevalence, severity, and correlates of problematic sexual internet use in Swedish men and women. Arch Sex Behav 41(2):459–466, 2012

Santos V, Freire R, Zugliani M, et al: Treatment outcomes in patients with internet addiction and anxiety. Medical Express 4(2):170–206, 2017

Schwartz MF, Southern S: Compulsive cybersex: the new tearoom. Sexual Addiction and Compulsivity 7:127–144, 2000

Siegel K, Meunier É, Lekas HM: Accounts for unprotected sex with partners met online from heterosexual men and women from large US metropolitan areas. AIDS Patient Care STDS 31(7):315–328, 2017

Sirianni JM, Vishwanath A: Problematic online pornography use: a media attendance perspective. J Sex Res 53(1):21–34, 2015

Snagowski J, Laier C, Duka T, Brand M: Subjective craving for pornography and associative learning predict tendencies towards cybersex addiction in a sample of regular cybersex users. Sexual Addiction and Compulsivity 23(4):342–360, 2016

Southern S: Treatment of compulsive cybersex behavior. Psychiatr Clin North Am 31:697–712, 2008

Spielberger CD, Gorsuch RL, Lushene RE: The State-Trait Anxiety Inventory Manual. Palo Alto, CA, Consulting Psychologists Press, 1970

Stark R, Kruse O, Snagowski J, et al: Predictors for (problematic) use of internet sexually explicit material: role of trait sexual motivation and implicit approach tendencies towards sexually explicit material. Sexual Addiction and Compulsivity 24(3):180–202, 2017

Stein DJ, Black DW, Shapira NA, Spitzer RL: Hypersexual disorder and preoccupation with internet pornography. Am J Psychiatry 158:1590–1594, 2001

Strasburger VC, Jordan AB, Donnerstein E: Children, adolescents, and the media: health effects. Pediatr Clin North Am 53(3):533–587, 2012

Twohig MP, Crosby JM: Acceptance and commitment therapy as a treatment for problematic internet pornography viewing. Behav Ther 41(3):285–295, 2010

Voon V, Mole TB, Banca P, et al: Neural correlates of sexual cue reactivity in individuals with and without compulsive sexual behaviours. PLoS One 9(7):e102419, 2014

Wéry A, Billieux J: Problematic cybersex: conceptualization, assessment, and treatment. Addict Behav 64:238–246, 2015

Wéry A, Billieux J: Online sexual activities: an exploratory study of problematic and non-problematic usage patterns in a sample of men. Comput Human Behav 56:257–266, 2016

Whitfield CL: Internal evidence and corroboration of traumatic memories of child sexual abuse with addictive disorders. Sexual Addiction and Compulsivity 5(4):269–292, 1998

World Health Organization: International Classification of Diseases and Related Health Problems, 11th Revision. Geneva, World Health Organization, 2019

Young KS: Internet sex addiction: risk factors, stages of development, and treatment. Am Behav Sci 52(1):21–37, 2008

CHAPTER 5

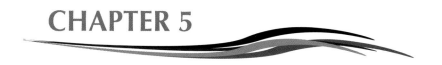

Diagnostic Aspects of CSBD

DSM AND BEYOND

Richard B. Krueger, M.D.

This chapter presents information on the diagnosis of hypersexual or compulsive sexual behavior in both the ICD-11 (World Health Organization 2020) and DSM-5 (American Psychiatric Association 2013), reviewing the utility and use of psychiatric diagnoses in general and their use in both diagnostic systems. The chapter then compares the ICD and DSM and discusses the advantages and disadvantages of each. Finally, it describes practical examples of cases involving sexual disorder diagnoses and summarizes the likely future usage of these diagnostic criteria.

DEFINITIONS AND UTILITY OF THE CONCEPT OF DIAGNOSIS

Nowhere in the various editions of DSM or ICD can one find a definition of the word or process of diagnosis. The *Oxford English Dictionary* definition of *diagnosis* is: "*Medicine*. Determination of the nature of a disease condition; identification of a disease by careful investigation of its symptoms and history; also, the opinion (formally stated) resulting from such investigation" (Oxford University Press 2019). *Diagnosis* comes from the Greek words for "distinguish, discern," "apart," and "recognize, know."

Psychiatric diagnoses have many uses. The World Psychiatric Association and the World Health Organization explored these in a survey of almost 5,000 psychiatrists using internet-based and printed interviews (G.M. Reed et al. 2011). They asked participants what they thought was the single most important purpose of a diagnostic classification system. Approximately 43% reported this as being for communication among clinicians, 27% for informing treatment and management decisions, 12% for communicating between clinicians and patients, 9% as a basis for generating national health statistics, 5% for research, and 4% for other purposes. Although 31% reported that, for maximum utility in clinical settings, a diagnostic manual should contain clear and strict criteria for all disorders, 69% indicated that they would prefer diagnostic guidance that was flexible enough to allow for cultural variation and clinical judgment, which was one of the main differences in the approach taken by ICD-10 (World Health Organization 1992) compared with DSM-IV-TR (American Psychiatric Association 2000; S.C. Reed et al. 2011), with ICD-10 being considered more flexible.

Overall, 70% of the global sample reported that ICD-10 was the classification system they used most in daily clinical work; 23% reported that they used DSM-IV (American Psychiatric Association 1994) most frequently; 6% reported using another classification system, such as the *Chinese Classification of Mental Disorders*, the *Cuban Glossary of Psychiatry*, or the *French Classification of Child and Adolescent Mental Disorders*, and 1% reported that they used ICD-9 or ICD-9-CM (S.C. Reed et al. 2011; U.S. Department of Health and Human Services 1989; World Health Organization 1975). Finally, 79% of participating psychiatrists (S.C. Reed et al. 2011), and, in a separate survey (Evans et al. 2013), 60% of psychologists reported that they often or almost always used a formal classification system in their everyday clinical work; 14% of psychiatrists and 18% of psychologists reported that they sometimes used one. Thus, mental health professionals use diagnostic classifications regularly, and a clear majority worldwide reported using ICD as compared with DSM.

INTERNATIONAL CLASSIFICATION OF DISEASES

ICD-6 Through ICD-10

The *International Classification of Diseases* has included terms that could refer to "pathological sexuality" since it first added a classification that included mental disorders in the ICD-6 in 1948 (World Health Organization 1948). The term *pathological sexuality* was included in ICD-6 and ICD-7 (World Health Organization 1955). This was changed to *unspecified sexual deviation* in ICD-8 (World Health Organization 1965), which included "pathological sexuality not otherwise specified." This category continued in ICD-9 (World Health Organization 1975) as "sexual deviation and disorders unspecified." The ICD-9 also developed coding, with some modifications specifically for use in the United States as was required in 1979, and this was published in 1989 as ICD-9-CM (Centers for Disease Control and Prevention 2019; U.S. Department of Health and Human Services 1989). This included the glossary definition of "unspecified psychosexual disorder," defined as "302.9 Other," which included nymphomania (i.e., uncontrollable or excessive sexual desire in a woman) and satyriasis (i.e., uncontrollable or excessive sexual desire in a man). The ICD-9-CM also listed "unspecified psychosexual disorder," which included "pathologic sexuality not otherwise specified" and "sexual deviation not otherwise specified." Neither of these editions had descriptions of the diagnostic criteria aside from these terms.

ICD-10 was the first edition to contain detailed descriptions of the various diagnostic criteria contained therein. In section F52, "Sexual Dysfunction Not Caused by Organic Disorder or Disease," the diagnosis of excessive sexual drive was used, which reflected dated and pejorative terminology (World Health Organization 1992, p. 194):

F52.7 Excessive sexual drive

Both men and women may occasionally complain of excessive sexual drive as a problem in its own right, usually during late teenage or early adulthood. When the excessive sexual drive is secondary to an affective disorder (F30–F39) or when it occurs during the early stages of dementia (F00–F03), the underlying disorder should be coded.

Includes: nymphomania satyriasis.

ICD-11

The diagnosis of "compulsive sexual behavior disorder" (CSBD) was suggested for inclusion in ICD-11 (Grant et al. 2014), removed from the chapter on sexual dysfunction and included in the chapter on impulse-control disorders. The proposed diagnostic guidelines were tested in international multilingual internet-based field studies using case material and field studies in clinical settings (Kraus et al. 2018). This study is currently in review. The current criteria from the impulse-control disorders section of the ICD-11 beta website are as follows (World Health Organization 2020):

6C72   Compulsive Sexual Behaviour Disorder

Essential (Required) Features:

A persistent pattern of failure to control intense, repetitive sexual impulses or urges resulting in repetitive sexual behaviour, manifested in one or more of the following:

- Engaging in repetitive sexual behaviour has become a central focus of the individual's life to the point of neglecting health and personal care or other interests, activities and responsibilities.
- The individual has made numerous unsuccessful efforts to control or significantly reduce repetitive sexual behaviour.
- The individual continues to engage in repetitive sexual behaviour despite adverse consequences (e.g., marital conflict due to sexual behaviour, financial or legal consequences, negative impact on health).

The pattern of failure to control intense, repetitive sexual impulses or urges and resulting repetitive sexual behaviour is manifested over an extended period of time (e.g., 6 months or more).

The pattern of failure to control intense, repetitive sexual impulses or urges and resulting repetitive sexual behaviour is not better accounted for by another mental disorder (e.g., Manic Episode) or other medical condition and is not due to the effect of a substance or medication.

The pattern of repetitive sexual behaviour results in marked distress or significant impairment in personal, family, social, educational, occupational, or other important areas of functioning. Distress that is entirely related to moral judgments and disapproval about sexual impulses, urges, or behaviours is not sufficient to meet this requirement.

The ICD-11 clinical descriptions and diagnostic guidelines contain information as to the boundary with normality and differential diagnosis, but this has not been made publicly available as of the present time. The ICD-11 was adopted in May 2019 and goes into effect in January 2022.

DIAGNOSTIC AND STATISTICAL MANUAL OF MENTAL DISORDERS

DSM-I Through DSM-IV-TR

The American Psychiatric Association's *Diagnostic and Statistical Manual of Mental Disorders* has contained terms that could refer to aberrant sexual behavior since it was first published in 1952. DSM-I (American Psychiatric Association 1952) had a category of "sexual deviation," with the notation that "This diagnosis is reserved for deviant sexuality which is not symptomatic of more extensive syndromes, such as schizophrenic and obsessional reactions" (p. 38) and without further description. DSM-II (American Psychiatric Association 1968) included 10 categories under the diagnosis "302 Sexual Deviations," one of which was "302.8 Other Sexual Deviation" and another "302.9 Unspecified Sexual Deviation." DSM-III (American Psychiatric Association 1980) included a chapter on psychosexual disorders in which the diagnosis of "302.89 Psychosexual Disorder Not Elsewhere Classified," defined as "a residual category for disorders whose chief manifestations are psychological disturbances related to sexuality not covered by any of the other specific categories in the diagnostic class of Psychosexual Disorders" (p. 282). It gave as an example "distress about a pattern of repeated sexual conquests with a succession of individuals who exist only as things to be used (Don Juanism and nymphomania)" (p. 283).

DSM-III-R (American Psychiatric Association 1987) included a chapter on sexual disorders that included "302.90 Sexual Disorder Not Otherwise Specified"—"Sexual Disorders that are not classifiable in any of the previous categories"—and listed as an example "distress about a pattern of repeated sexual conquests or other forms of nonparaphilic sexual addiction, involving a succession of people who exist only as things to be used" (p. 296). DSM-IV continued with the catchall category of "302.9 Sexual Disorder Not Otherwise Specified," with an example similar to those in previous editions: "Distress about a pattern of repeated sexual relationships involving a succession of lovers who are experienced by the individual only as things to be used" (p. 538). DSM-IV-TR made no changes to this diagnosis.

DSM-5

The Paraphilic Disorders Subcommittee of the DSM-5 Work Group on Sexual and Gender Identity Disorders tasked with reviewing and updat-

Table 5–1.   Proposed diagnostic criteria for hypersexual disorder

A. Over a period of at least 6 months, recurrent and intense sexual fantasies, sexual urges, or sexual behaviors in association with three or more of the following five criteria:

   A1. Time consumed by sexual fantasies, urges or behaviors repetitively interferes with other important (non-sexual) goals, activities, and obligations.

   A2. Repetitively engaging in sexual fantasies, urges or behaviors in response to dysphoric mood states (e.g., anxiety, depression, boredom, irritability).

   A3. Repetitively engaging in sexual fantasies, urges or behaviors in response to stressful life events.

   A4. Repetitive but unsuccessful efforts to control or significantly reduce these sexual fantasies, urges or behaviors.

   A5. Repetitively engaging in sexual behaviors while disregarding the risk for physical or emotional harm to self or others.

B. There is clinically significant personal distress or impairment in social, occupational or other important areas of functioning associated with the frequency and intensity of these sexual fantasies, urges or behaviors.

C. These sexual fantasies, urges or behaviors are not due to the direct physiological effect of an exogenous substance (e.g., a drug of abuse or medication).

Specify if:
   Masturbation
   Pornography
   Sexual Behavior With Consenting Adults
   Cybersex
   Telephone Sex
   Strip Clubs
   Other

Source.   Kafka 2010, p. 379.

ing the diagnostic criteria for paraphilic disorders for DSM-5 also considered the possibility of developing diagnostic criteria for a diagnosis of hypersexual disorder (HD). Drawing from the review and suggestions of Stein et al. (2000), the subgroup proposed diagnostic criteria for HD (Table 5–1) and suggested including it in the section on "Conditions for Further Study."

The American Psychiatric Association's Board of Trustees ultimately rejected this recommendation. The reasons for the rejection were the insufficient scientific evidence that the proposed criteria in fact represented a distinct clinical syndrome and the concern that the diagnosis of

HD could potentially be misused in forensic settings (Kafka 2014). This left clinicians in a quandary as to how to diagnose a person with hypersexual behavior, given that the residual category in DSM-IV designated for such cases, sexual disorder not otherwise specified, had been removed from DSM-5 (Kafka 2014).

When ICD-10-CM was initially prepared in the 1990s, the diagnostic code of "F52.7 Excessive Sexual Drive" was decommissioned for use in the United States as part of an effort to have ICD-10-CM only include mental disorders that were also included in DSM-IV (American Medical Association 2016). According to the ICD-10-CM index, the diagnostic code that corresponded to "excessive sexual drive" was F52.8, "Other Sexual Dysfunction Not Due to Substance or Known Physiological Condition" (American Medical Association 2016; Krueger 2016). The ICD-10-CM index also included the terms *erotomania*, *nymphomania*, and *satyriasis* and indexed them to F52.8 as well, reflecting their historical use referring to excessive sexual drive. Such terms are obviously pejorative and unlikely to be used by clinicians.

DSM-5 lists diagnoses of "Other Specified Sexual Dysfunction 302.79 (F52.8)" and "Unspecified Sexual Dysfunction 302.70 (F52.9)." Given that hypersexuality is not a sexual dysfunction per se, both it (and its historically related terms) are not given as examples under the DSM-5 category of other specified sexual dysfunction. Similarly, because it is not a paraphilia, the residual code for other specified paraphilic disorder would also not be appropriate. One category used by clinicians to diagnose cases of hypersexual or compulsive sexual behavior is "Other Specified Disruptive, Impulse-Control, and Conduct Disorder 312.89 (F91.8)." The specific definition of this category appears in Box 5–1.

Box 5–1.   Other Specified Disruptive, Impulse-Control, and Conduct Disorder 312.89 (F91.8)

This category applies to presentations in which symptoms characteristic of a disruptive, impulse-control, and conduct disorder that cause clinically significant distress or impairment in social, occupational, or other important areas of functioning predominate but do not meet the full criteria for any of the disorders in the disruptive, impulse-control, and conduct disorders diagnostic class. The other specified disruptive, impulse-control, and conduct disorder category is used in situations in which the clinician chooses to communicate the specific reason that the presentation does not meet the criteria for any specific disruptive, impulse-control, and conduct disorder. This is done by recording "other specified disruptive, impulse-control, and conduct disorder" followed by the specific reason (e.g., "recurrent behavioral outbursts of insufficient frequency").

> ### Box 5–2.   Other Specified Mental Disorder 300.9 (F99)
>
> This category applies to presentations in which symptoms characteristic of a mental disorder that cause clinically significant distress or impairment in social, occupational, or other important areas of functioning predominate but do not meet the full criteria for any specific mental disorder. The other specified mental disorder category is used in situations in which the clinician chooses to communicate the specific reason that the presentation does not meet the criteria for any specific mental disorder. This is done by recording "other specified mental disorder" followed by the specific reason.

Thus, if one considers hypersexuality or compulsive sexual behavior a disturbance in impulse control, this category would be the most appropriate diagnosis in DSM-5, which is consistent with the placement of CSBD within the impulse-control disorders in the ICD-11 (Reed et al. 2019). Clinicians would record this diagnosis as "F52.8, Other Specified Disruptive, Impulse-Control, and Conduct Disorder, Hypersexuality" and write the specific reason why this category is being used as opposed to a more specific category. This reasoning would require elaboration of more specific criteria or reasons from sources other than DSM-5, because no diagnostic category or guidance for hypersexual or compulsive sexual behavior exists in DSM-5 to explain why the particular disorder does not meet the usual criteria; for example, a clinician might write, "patient has a pattern of compulsive or hypersexual behavior involving sexual behavior which is distressing and interfering with his or her functioning." Because no description of hypersexual behavior appears anywhere in DSM-5, clinicians would have to rely on other sources, including prior editions of DSM, definitions from the literature, or, perhaps, because it will be authoritative and available, the definition from ICD-11.

Another possible way of diagnosing HD or CSBD in DSM-5 would be to use the more broadly defined diagnosis of "Other Specified Mental Disorder 300.9 (F99)." The description of this diagnosis is presented in Box 5–2. The disadvantage to this is that insurance companies do not favor diagnoses at such a high level of abstraction; in addition, such diagnoses may not as readily convey more specific information needed for care or communication among providers and provide no information that would be of use epidemiologically. Another issue with diagnoses that include specific reference to hypersexual or compulsive sexual behavior is that of clinicians not wanting to stigmatize their patients with such a diagnosis. Survey information in the United States from a National Ambulatory Medical Care survey of more than 400,000,000 visits to various medical care providers recorded no visits with the diagnoses of sexual sadism or sexual masochism (Krueger 2010). This absence may reflect providers' concerns about stigmatizing patients with these diagnoses, as well as an absence of patients treated for these diagnoses. It may also reflect the practice of listing other diagnoses, such as depression or anxiety, as the primary reason for the visit; often providers will opt to do this instead of including diagnoses they consider stigmatizing.

COMPARISON OF ICD WITH DSM

The ICD and DSM have often been compared, and sexual disorders have been included in such comparisons. First (2009) reported in a study comparing ICD-10 with DSM-IV-TR that, considering the sexual disorders, the only category in which there was a conceptual difference between DSM and ICD definitions was gender identity disorder. While this study also noted differences in the DSM-IV-TR and ICD-10 definitions of the paraphilias and sexual disorders, these were considered to be only in wording and not representative of a conceptual difference between the manuals. Table 5–2 summarizes some of the differences between the ICD and DSM.

Overall, a significant number of differences exist in terms of the development, usage, and mandate between ICD and DSM. The United States is required to use ICD codes for reporting health statistics as a result of its being a signatory on a United Nations document. The government agency responsible for implementing ICD in the United States is the National Center for Health Statistics (NCHS), which is part of the Centers for Disease Control and Prevention. Codes are approved by a joint group called the ICD-CM Coordination and Maintenance Committee, which is made up of representatives of NCHS, the Centers for Medicare and Medicaid Services, and the American Hospital Association. Although modified forms of ICD-10 codes were adopted for usage in the United States in 2016, most of the rest of the world adopted its usage shortly after publication of ICD-10 in 1992. The reason for the delay in adopting ICD codes in the United States involved resistance by medical and hospital communities to the cost of converting from ICD-9-CM to ICD-10-CM.

CASE EXAMPLES

The following examples are compilations from a number of patients but accurately represent archetypal clinical examples encountered in real practice.

Table 5–2.   Comparison of ICD and DSM

ICD	DSM
Produced and published by the World Health Organization, the global health agency of the United Nations	Produced and published by a single national professional association, the American Psychiatric Association (APA)
Free and open resource to advance the public good and improve the health of all people	Provides a large portion of revenues for the APA
For countries and front-line services providers	Developed mainly for psychiatrists and mental health professionals; can also be used by primary care and other providers
Global, multidisciplinary, multilingual development	Dominated by the United States and anglophone perspective
Approved by the World Health Assembly	Approved by the APA Board of Trustees
Covers all health conditions	Covers only mental disorders
Published in 2019	Most recent edition published in 2013, with periodic updates since then
Priority and criteria for change involve clinical utility and reducing the disease burden of the countries of the world	Priority and criteria for change involve scientific justification or correction for modification
Use of manual and diagnostic codes agreed to by international treaty by all parties	No broad governmental mandate for use; usage requirement determined by specific agencies or entities
Stylistically described as consisting of prototypical narratives	Stylistically described as consisting of iterations of specific diagnostic criteria

Mr. K

Mr. K was a 35-year-old single male who lived alone in a studio apartment. He had been raised in the orthodox Jewish religion, but he had stopped practicing many years earlier. He had a college education and had worked as a waiter and at the front desks of hotels until he was disabled by a work injury several years before he came for an evaluation.

With his disability, he had spent increasing amounts of time in his apartment. He had become depressed and anxious and had seen a psychopharmacologist for evaluation for possible medication treatment and then seen a therapist weekly. He was diagnosed as having claustrophobia, anxiety, and depression and was treated with buspirone and sertraline, with some improvement in his symptoms. He was referred for an evaluation for "out of control sexual behavior."

Sexually, he had realized that he had a gay orientation since he was prepubertal and over many years had engaged in brief relationships with men whom he met, often with unsafe sexual behavior. Of more concern to him were his masturbatory habits and other "compulsive" sexual behaviors. He said that since he had been on disability, he would look at pornography and engage in cybersexual interactions constantly, engage in telephone sex, which he could not afford, and masturbate throughout the day. He had an average of 35 ejaculations per week. He thought that this sexual behavior interfered with his ability to find employment and get off of disability and that it also interfered with his ability to engage in sexual relationships with men. He had attended 12-step "sexaholic" meetings for several months, which were not helpful, and he thought the sertraline and buspirone had had no effect on his sexual interest or outlet. He said he had zero control over his sexual behavior.

Mr. K was diagnosed according to DSM-IV-TR as having a sexual disorder not otherwise specified. He also received diagnoses of major depression, recurrent, and anxiety disorder not otherwise specified. He was treated with depot leuprolide acetate, and over the next 6 months he reduced his ejaculatory frequency to twice per month. He stopped engaging in cybersex and telephone sex and markedly reduced his use of pornography. He was extremely pleased with his response to this medication, saying, "I finally got control over my sexual behavior." His depot leuprolide acetate was discontinued after a total of 6 months of treatment, and on follow-up at 1 year he was still not masturbating (a goal established in 12-step meetings) and was fully employed. He continued with 12-step groups for sexaholics and had resumed sexual relationships with men. He was no longer depressed.

We can see that Mr. K's symptoms fulfilled virtually all of the criteria for HD as recommended by the DSM-5 Work Group and for CSBD according to ICD-11. Unfortunately, his diagnosis according to DSM-5 criteria would be other specified disruptive, impulse-control, and conduct disorder. Although information concerning the basis for this diagnosis would be written in by the provider, such information would have to rely on a definition of hypersexual or compulsive sexual behavior not found in DSM-5. Accordingly, a clinician would have to rely on other information for guidance to make such a diagnosis, such as that presented in the literature (Kaplan and Krueger 2010) or from ICD-10 or ICD-11.

Mr. L

Mr. L was a 40-year-old male raised in the Protestant religion who was married but had moved away from his wife after she discovered that she had contracted herpes from him. He worked in the computer industry. He was intellectually gifted and very successful in his career. He and his wife had been married for 3 years but had fought often because of his use of pornography and masturbation. He said that he had been hypersexual for many years. Mr. L was heterosexual in his sexual orientation.

He said that during puberty he began masturbating frequently. After marriage, he began engaging in sexual behavior with women other than his wife when he was away on business, frequently engaging in unprotected sex. He denied any paraphilic behavior. He acknowledged masturbating to pornography up to 8–10 hours per day, to the point that he would injure his penis. He had no prior history of mental health treatment. He also was significantly depressed.

Mr. L was diagnosed with major depression, single episode, and sexual disorder not otherwise specified, characterized by pornography dependence, masturbation, and sexual behavior involving adults. He was treated with sertraline, and his depression improved. He engaged in individual therapy for his hypersexual behavior for a brief period of time, and initially, his control over his sexual behavior improved. However, eventually he resumed acting out sexually, even though his depression was treated, and he and his wife separated. He refused other treatment recommendations for his hypersexual behavior.

Again the patient could be diagnosed using DSM-5 criteria for other specified disruptive, impulse-control, and conduct disorder. Given that the ICD-10 codes for such hypersexual behavior, including excessive sexual drive, other sexual dysfunction not caused by organic disorder or disease, and unspecified sexual dysfunction not caused by organic disorder or disease, are associated with the pejorative diagnosis, it would seem that the appropriate diagnosis in the United States according to the ICD-10 would be other conduct disorders (F91.8). In other countries, Mr. L could be diagnosed with excessive sexual drive.

The ICD-11 was adopted in 2019, but it does not go into effect until 2022. One could anticipate, given its prior history of delayed adoption of such criteria, that the United States will take many years before adopting the ICD-11 classification for official use. However, the lack of specificity of any diagnoses in DSM-5 for hypersexual or compulsive sexual behavior and the use of an alternative broad diagnosis of other specified disruptive, impulse-control, and conduct disorder will likely result in the ICD-11 criteria for CSBD being used by clinicians to further describe their use of this diagnosis.

SUMMARY AND CONCLUSION

Diagnostic names and codes for hypersexual or compulsive sexual behavior have been included in the World Health Organization's *International Classification of Diseases* since it began listing mental disorders with the ICD-6 in 1948, and they have been included in the American Psychiatric Association's *Diagnostic and Statistical Manual of Mental Disorders* since its inception in 1952. Both the ICD-10 and DSM-IV-TR contained codes and some diagnostic criteria and other information that referred to hypersexual or compulsive sexual behavior. However, although the code and diagnostic criteria for this entity have been continued in the ICD-11, they were discontinued in DSM-5. It is possible that DSM could include a diagnosis similar to the ICD-11's CSBD, but none has been adopted as yet, and inclusion will require significant effort with substantial scientific support. Alternative diagnoses that can be used in DSM-5 currently include other specified disruptive, impulse-control, and conduct disorder and other specified mental disorder, although there are no specifications for the diagnostic criteria within DSM-5. Other sources, such as the literature, prior diagnostic suggestions, or the definitions in the ICD-11 would need to be used to provide such specification. Although the ICD-11 may not be accepted for use in the United States for many years, its criteria for CSBD are available and, it can be anticipated, will be used to support the substitute diagnoses in DSM-5. Clinicians outside of the United States may start using the new ICD-11 criteria when their individual countries decide to adopt it, with each country doing this in their own time frame.

It might be argued that the ICD-11 codes may not be used in the United States until the ICD-11 is officially adopted, but, clearly, acceptable substitute codes in DSM-5 could be used immediately. Even from the perspective of forensic psychiatry, the fact that the ICD-11 is available, with all of its supporting literature, makes it likely that it will rapidly be considered authoritative, even though it and its codes may not be formally accepted. Finally, it is unfortunate that it took so long for the United States to accept the ICD-10, resulting in the loss of a significant stream of epidemiological and diagnostic data, and it is hoped that adoption of the ICD-11 will take less time. Adoption of the ICD-11 criteria in the United States and elsewhere could also afford significant opportunities for the evaluation of these criteria and facilitate research into the more basic aspects of hypersexual behavior (Briken and Krueger 2018).

REFERENCES

American Medical Association: ICD-10-CM: The Complete Official Draft Code Set. Evanston, IL, American Medical Association, 2016

American Psychiatric Association: Diagnostic and Statistical Manual: Mental Disorders. Washington, DC, American Psychiatric Association, 1952

American Psychiatric Association: Diagnostic and Statistical Manual of Mental Disorders, 2nd Edition. Washington, DC, American Psychiatric Association, 1968

American Psychiatric Association: Diagnostic and Statistical Manual of Mental Disorders, 3rd Edition. Washington, DC, American Psychiatric Association, 1980

American Psychiatric Association: Diagnostic and Statistical Manual of Mental Disorders, 3rd Edition, Revised. Washington, DC, American Psychiatric Association, 1987

American Psychiatric Association: Diagnostic and Statistical Manual of Mental Disorders, 4th Edition. Washington, DC, American Psychiatric Association, 1994

American Psychiatric Association: Diagnostic and Statistical Manual of Mental Disorders, 4th Edition, Text Revision. Washington, DC, American Psychiatric Association, 2000

American Psychiatric Association: Diagnostic and Statistical Manual of Mental Disorders, 5th Edition. Arlington, VA, American Psychiatric Association, 2013

Briken P, Krueger RB: From atypical sexual interests to paraphilic disorders: the planned ICD revisions related to paraphilic disorder. J Sex Med 15:807–808, 2018

Centers for Disease Control and Prevention: International Classification of Diseases, 9th Revision. Atlanta, GA, Centers for Disease Control and Prevention, 2019

Evans SC, Reed GM, Roberts MC, et al: Psychologists' perspectives on the diagnostic classification of mental disorders: results from the WHO-IUPsyS Global Survey. Int J Psychol 48(3):177–193, 2013

First MB: Harmonisation of ICD-11 and DSM-V: opportunities and challenges. Br J Psychiatry 195:382–390, 2009

Grant JE, Atmaca M, Fineberg NA, et al: Impulse control disorders and behavioural addictions in the ICD-11. World Psychiatry 13(2):125–127, 2014

Kafka MP: Hypersexual disorder: a proposed diagnosis for DSM-V. Arch Sex Behav 39(2):377–400, 2010

Kafka MP: What happened to hypersexual disorder? Arch Sex Behav 43(7):1259–1261, 2014

Kaplan MS, Krueger RB: Diagnosis, assessment, and treatment of hypersexuality. J Sex Res 47(2–3):181–198, 2010

Kraus SW, Krueger RB, Briken P, et al: Compulsive sexual behaviour disorder in the ICD-11. World Psychiatry 17(1):109–110, 2018

Krueger RB: The DSM diagnostic criteria for sexual sadism. Arch Sex Behav 39(2):325–345, 2010

Krueger RB: Diagnosis of hypersexual or compulsive sexual behavior can be made using ICD-10 and DSM-5 despite rejection of this diagnosis by the American Psychiatric Association. Addiction 111:2107–2114, 2016

Oxford University Press: Oxford English Dictionary. New York, Oxford University Press, 2019

Reed GM, Correia JM, Esparza P, et al: The WPA-WHO global survey of psychiatrist's attitudes toward mental disorders classification. World Psychiatry 10(2):118–131, 2011

Reed GM, First MB, Kogan CS, et al: Innovations and changes in the ICD-11 classification of mental, behavioural and neurodevelopmental disorders. World Psychiatry 18:1–18, 2019

Reed SC, Evans SM, Bedi G, et al: The effects of oral micronized progesterone on smoked cocaine self-administration in women. Horm Behav 59, 227–235, 2011

U.S. Department of Health and Human Services: International Classification of Diseases, 9th Revision, Clinical Modification, 3rd Edition, Vol 1. Washington, DC, U.S. Dept. of Health and Human Services, 1989

not simply a result of rejection or feared rejection of the arousal pattern by others or with significant risk of injury or death. (World Health Organization 2019)

Paraphilic behaviors are those considered to be outside the conventional range of sexual behaviors. Paraphilias often begin during late adolescence and peak in the mid-20s. Nonparaphilic behaviors (e.g., sex with multiple partners, constant sexual fixation on an unattainable partner, compulsive masturbation, attendance at strip clubs, and compulsive use of pornography) may be subsumed under the CSBD diagnosis and are consensual sexual practices. The onset, clinical course, and male predominance of nonparaphilic behaviors are similar to those of paraphilic disorders.

HYPERSEXUAL DISORDER

HD is a pattern of recurrent intense and excessive preoccupation with sexual fantasies, urges, and behavior that individuals struggle to control (Kafka 2010; Reid et al. 2011). It has been described as an "inability to regulate one's sexual behavior that is a source of significant personal distress" (Walton et al. 2017). Clinically, HD includes symptoms such as a high frequency of sexual activity, subjective symptoms (perceiving one's sexual behavior as uncontrollable), and adverse life consequences such as sexually transmitted infections, unplanned pregnancies, relationship conflict and dissolution, social isolation, loss of employment, legal violations, and indebtedness (Reid et al. 2010, 2012). The DSM-5 Work Group on Sexual and Gender Identity Disorders recommended diagnostic criteria for HD (Table 6–1). Like CSBD, HD was primarily conceptualized as a nonparaphilic sexual desire disorder driven by impulsivity (Kafka 2001). Although field trials conducted by the DSM-5 Work Group showed that the criteria were reliable (Reid et al. 2012), CSBD was not included in the DSM-5 classification (American Psychiatric Association 2013) for at least the following two reasons: 1) insufficient scientific evidence that the proposed diagnostic criteria represented a distinct clinical disorder; and 2) the potential misuse of the HD diagnosis in clinical and especially forensic settings (Kafka 2014).

SEXUAL ADDICTION

The diagnosis of SA posits that problematic, uncontrollable sexual behaviors stem from a behavioral addiction (Birchard 2011; Carnes 1992). SA does not exclude paraphilias, and therefore the symptoms of SA may

---

Table 6–1.   Proposed diagnostic criteria for hypersexual disorder

A. Over a period of at least 6 months, recurrent and intense sexual fantasies, sexual urges, or sexual behaviors in association with three or more of the following five criteria:

   A1. Time consumed by sexual fantasies, urges or behaviors repetitively interferes with other important (non-sexual) goals, activities, and obligations.

   A2. Repetitively engaging in sexual fantasies, urges or behaviors in response to dysphoric mood states (e.g., anxiety, depression, boredom, irritability).

   A3. Repetitively engaging in sexual fantasies, urges or behaviors in response to stressful life events.

   A4. Repetitive but unsuccessful efforts to control or significantly reduce these sexual fantasies, urges or behaviors.

   A5. Repetitively engaging in sexual behaviors while disregarding the risk for physical or emotional harm to self or others.

B. There is clinically significant personal distress or impairment in social, occupational or other important areas of functioning associated with the frequency and intensity of these sexual fantasies, urges or behaviors.

C. These sexual fantasies, urges or behaviors are not due to the direct physiological effect of an exogenous substance (e.g., a drug of abuse or medication).

Specify if:
   Masturbation
   Pornography
   Sexual Behavior With Consenting Adults
   Cybersex
   Telephone Sex
   Strip Clubs
   Other

Source.   Kafka 2010, p. 379.

---

involve paraphiliac behaviors such as fetishism or pedophilia. However, most practicing SA clinicians do not assess or treat patients who are sexual offenders and are diagnosed with paraphilias such as pedophilia.

Carnes and Wilson (2002) and others have conceptualized SA as the result of deep emotional pain associated with child abuse and trauma, comorbid physical and mental health problems, and a history of family addiction. More recently, researchers and theorists have proposed that SA is driven by dysfunctional attachment, impaired impulse control, shame, and mood disorders (Riemersma and Sytsma 2013) and is maintained by obsession, sexual triggers and rituals, CSB, and emotional despair consistent with a wounded sense of self. Other defining features of SA are obsession or preoccupation with obtaining, using, or recovering from the behavior, loss of control (e.g., persistent desire or unsuccessful efforts to curtail the behavior), and continuing the behavior despite adverse consequences (Carnes and Schneider 2000).

Models suggest that SA is a combination of a desire for pleasure production and an aversion to pain that is characterized by recurrent failure to control one's sexual behaviors and continuation of sexual behavior despite substantial harmful consequences (Goodman 1998). Goodman (1998) suggested that SA involves impairment of three neurobiological systems—1) reward motivation, 2) affect regulation, and 3) behavioral inhibition—and delineated criteria for SA as shown in Table 6–2. SA involves intense sexual craving that is both psychological and physiological (Grant et al. 2014). Carnes's criteria for SA are shown in Table 6–3 and apply the criteria traditionally associated with substance use disorders (SUDs), such as dependence and tolerance (Carnes 2000).

CLINICAL ASSESSMENT OF COMPULSIVE SEXUAL BEHAVIOR DISORDER

Although assessment of problematic sexual behavior should include a structured clinical interview, routine medical screening, use of psychometric testing, and collateral assessment information from family members or partner(s) when appropriate, the central and most important part of the clinical assessment of CSBD is the clinical interview.

Clinical Interview

Patients with problematic sex behaviors are typically not candid about their situation or problem and may not even recognize that it *is* a problem (Carnes and Wilson 2002). Patients often come to an assessment because of pressure from a partner, friends, or family members; because of an entanglement with the law; or because their problem has come to the attention of their employer. Clinicians should be aware that when patients hold a position of leadership or power (e.g., in their church, their business, their community, or politics), they may have a sound motivation for withholding information regarding divergent sexual behavior. Assessment might also be obscured by a convoluted marital or employment situation for which the patient may have successfully avoided visible consequences thus far. Thus, the clinician may have little initial information from which to draw an accurate clinical conclusion.

Table 6–2.   Goodman's sexual addiction criteria

A maladaptive pattern of sexual behavior leading to clinically significant impairment or distress, as manifested by three (or more) of the following, occurring at any time in the same 12-month period:

1. Tolerance, as defined by either of the following:

   a. Need for markedly increased amount or intensity of the sexual behavior to achieve the desired effect.

   b. Markedly diminished effect with continued involvement in the sexual behavior at the same level of intensity.

2. Withdrawal, as manifested by either of the following:

   a. Characteristic psychophysiological withdrawal syndrome of physiologically described changes and/or psychologically described changes upon discontinuation of the sexual behavior.

   b. Engagement in the same (or a closely related) sexual behavior to relieve or avoid withdrawal symptoms.

3. Sexual behavior is often engaged in over a longer period, in greater quantity, or at a higher level of intensity than intended.

4. There is a persistent desire or unsuccessful efforts to cut down or control the sexual behavior.

5. A great deal of time is spent on activities necessary to prepare for the sexual behavior, engage in the behavior, or recover from its effects.

6. Important social, occupational, or recreational activities are given up or reduced because of the sexual behavior.

7. The sexual behavior continues despite knowledge of having a persistent or recurrent physical or psychological problem that is likely to have been caused or exacerbated by the behavior.

Source.   Adapted from Goodman 1998.

A structured interview offers both formality and flexibility, letting patients discuss their experiences using their own descriptive words and meanings. It is important for clinicians to pay attention to behaviors such as avoidance, emotional detachment, and minimization because patients often minimize the extent of their problems. Collateral assessment information, such as reports from partners, family, and friends; medical records; and court documents, may provide data that are not observable under other assessment conditions, but these may be difficult to gather.

The first step when evaluating any psychiatric patient is a thorough standard psychiatric assessment. Such an evaluation should begin with an interview performed by a psychiatrist or clinical psychologist to assess the history of the current complaint, any psychological and physi-

---

Table 6–3. Carnes' sexual addiction criteria

A. A minimum of three criteria met during a 12-month period:

1. Recurrent failure to resist impulses to engage in specific sexual behavior

2. Frequent engaging in these behaviors to a greater extent or longer duration than intended

3. Persistent desire or unsuccessful efforts to stop, to reduce, or to control behaviors

4. Inordinate amount of time spent in obtaining sex, being sexual, or recovering from sexual experiences

5. Preoccupation with the behavior or preparatory activities

6. Frequent engaging in the behavior when expected to fulfill occupational, academic, domestic, or social obligations

7. Continuation of the behavior despite knowledge of having a persistent or recurrent social, financial, psychological, or physical problem that is caused or exacerbated by the behavior

8. Need to increase intensity, frequency, number, or risk of behaviors to achieve the desired effect or diminished effect with continued behaviors at the same level of intensity, frequency, number, or risk

9. Giving up or limiting social, occupational, or recreational activities because of behavior

10. Distress, anxiety, restlessness, or irritability if unable to engage in the behaviors

B. Has significant personal and social consequences (such as loss of partner, occupation, or legal implications)

Source. Carnes 2000.

---

cal stressors, a full psychosocial history, and routine medical tests to rule out any contributory or causative medical conditions. The examination should include a sexual status examination that—akin to a mental status examination that assesses a patient's mental state—describes sexual encounters and understands the patient's states of desire, arousal, and orgasm. The examiner should have experience in sensitively taking a sexual history that provides an accurate portrait of the person's sexual activity, arousal template, likes and dislikes, and desires and inhibitions in order to fully appreciate the frequency and nature of the person's sexual problem(s) (Bartlik et al. 2013).

During the initial interview, it is important to acquire as much information as possible about the patient's sexual behaviors. Clinicians should ask questions about the patient's sexual history, family of origin, and experiences growing up. To begin exploring the patient's sexually compulsive symptoms, clinicians might consider asking questions from the simple screening method known as PATHOS (Carnes et al. 2012):

P—Do you often find yourself **P**reoccupied with sexual thoughts?
A—Do you hide some of your sexual behaviors from others (because you feel **A**shamed)?
T—Have you ever sought **T**reatment or other help for your sexual behavior?
H—Has anyone been **H**urt emotionally because of your sexual behavior?
O—Do you feel controlled by your sexual behavior, or that your sex life is **O**ut of control?
S—When you have sex, do you feel depressed or **S**ad afterward?

Each positively answered item results in one point. The PATHOS is not a verified psychometric assessment; however, using a cutoff score of 3 points or higher, our experience is that the PATHOS is a good clinical indicator that further exploration of the patient's sexual behavior is needed. It is also a useful starting point for the in-depth portion of the clinical interview. When patients respond affirmatively to one or more questions, clinicians can ask for more information, which can open the lines of communication regarding sexual issues. The information elicited from both general questioning about sex and sexuality and from a PATHOS screening is a good introduction to more specific inquiry about issues related to hypersexuality.

Acquiring an accurate history of a patient's behaviors may be difficult during the clinical interview for various reasons, such as the patient's marital status or status in the community or the societal norms regarding inappropriate sexual behavior. The patient's situation, shame, or even lack of awareness of a problem may severely limit a clinician's access to needed information. As a result, disclosure can be slow, and the clinician is unlikely to get the whole story in the initial session. Moreover, as we see with other disorders of addiction, individuals with problematic sexual behaviors often engage in distorted thinking—defending, justifying, and blaming others for their problems. Many deny that they have a problem and seek help only to appease an angry spouse or to avoid criminal prosecution. Additionally, persons with probable CSBD are adept at presenting themselves in favorable ways, often by not disclosing problematic behaviors beyond their presenting issue and minimizing or even denying problematic behaviors. They might also disclose past behaviors while hiding current problems. Denial, avoidance, and minimization are common, compounded by the typical beliefs patients have at this stage of engagement, including the thoughts that nothing will help them, that everything will be fine if they decrease their sexual misbehavior, or that they are only in therapy to appease a relative, the law, or a spouse.

We find it may be useful to normalize patients' difficulty by explaining that it is common to hold back information and that many people with these problems do not fully realize the impact their compulsion has had on their lives (and on the people around them) until they begin uncovering their compulsive or addictive behaviors. In such cases, asking for more specific details during the disclosure process, such as how many times a day the patient masturbates or how many hours the patient spends looking at pornography each day, can help the patient recognize patterns of CSBD, as well as ongoing denial. Key questions in the clinical interview assessment are shown in Table 6–4.

Many times, denial operates without conscious awareness, leaving patients largely unaware of the entirety of their maladaptive patterns. Such patients may compartmentalize their thinking in ways that prevent them from recognizing and examining their behavior and its consequences. Patients might also be so anxious about consequences, such as an impending court date or a divorce, that they may not remember certain details of the sexual acting out—that is, their anxiety overrides their memory.

Needless to say, disclosure is usually a slow process, but as the therapeutic alliance builds, patients begin to feel safe enough to tell their stories, including their most painful and shameful things. Clinicians must be patient with this process, because patients may require titration to digest their experiences without being overwhelmed. Clinicians must also query patients about nonproblematic sexual behaviors with partners, using a current sexual status examination that details "normal," nonproblematic or noncompulsive sexual behaviors.

As we discuss in the sections that follow, interviewers should consider contributing, comorbid, and collateral issues. Many people with addiction issues are genetically predisposed (Blum et al. 2014; Goldman et al. 2005; Kreek et al. 2005) and may have a family history of substance abuse or compulsive behaviors. Individuals with problematic sexual behaviors often have a history of intimacy issues in romantic relationships and may also have other life challenges, such as family issues or other types of clinical disorders. Exposure to sexually explicit information (e.g., stories with sexual content, pornography, sexual acts) as a child may also be a contributing factor.

CSBD may be associated with difficulties with normative sexual and romantic intimacy. In our experience, as individuals with CSBD fever-

Table 6–4. Clinical interview assessment of patients with compulsive sexual behavior disorder (CSBD)

Key question	Common feature in CSBD
Do you often find yourself preoccupied or consumed with sexual thoughts or behaviors to an extent that is distressing or out of bounds compared with your peers?	Preoccupation with sex, spending considerable time fantasizing about, procuring, and planning sexual experiences to an extent that is extreme compared with peers
Do you hide your deepest sexual desires or behaviors from others, and do you frequently engage in sexual behaviors that you later regret or feel ashamed of?	Exceptional hiding, lowered self-esteem, and shame about thoughts and actions that is well beyond person's own barometer of acceptable behavior
Do you feel controlled by your sexual desires or behaviors and feel that your sex life is completely out of control?	Vulnerability or loss of control in engaging in sexual experiences to a far greater extent than intended
Have your problematic sexual desires or actions increased in frequency and the associated level of risk taking?	Tolerance or a need for more intense experiences to get aroused
Do your sexual thoughts or behaviors consume significant portions of your available time or financial resources?	Inordinate losses of personal time and finances spent on planning and executing sexual escapades
Do your sexual thoughts or behaviors interfere with and preempt time with work, friends, family, and healthy relationships (as you would define "healthy relationships")?	Significant and severe interference with their occupational and social functioning as a consequence of sexual thoughts and behaviors

ishly pursue their dysfunctional sexual behaviors, they may have difficulties with their intimate partners, healthy sexual encounters, or stable relationships. These difficulties may, in part, have motivated or risen as a consequence of the CSBD. Premature ejaculation, erectile dysfunction, anorgasmia, and extended periods during which the person has no sexual activity are commonly seen in this clinical population and need to be pursued in the sexual status examination. Psychological stressors are associated with CSBD. Anecdotally, the first author (K.P.R.) has observed the onset of CSBD in patients following the death of a close relative and other psychological stressors. Stress itself can be an inducer or a consequence of sexual compulsivity, and an association exists between exaggerated physiological stress responses and hypersexuality (Chatzittofis et al. 2016).

Table 6–5. Disorders commonly presenting with compulsive sexual behavior disorder (CSBD)-like behaviors

Bipolar disorder, mania, or hypomania	Compulsive sexuality can be a symptom of other disorders, particularly frontal brain syndromes and psychiatric disorders such as mania. This is especially the case if CSBD symptoms appear *only* during acute illness or, in the case of substance abuse disorders, during intoxication.
Frontal or temporal lesions, Parkinson's disease, dementias	
Personality disorder: especially borderline pattern	
Substance abuse disorders: particularly stimulant abuse	Neuropsychiatric disorders may frequently be comorbid with the diagnosis of CSBD, particularly mood disorders, anxiety disorders, personality disorders with a borderline patterns, substance abuse, autism, and paraphilias.
Autism spectrum disorders	
ADHD	
Paraphilias	

Assessment of Co-Occurring Disorders

A skillful, structured psychiatric interview needs to rule out other psychiatric disorders that may be associated with sexual hyperactivity, such as bipolar disorder, OCD, substance abuse, psychotic disorders, and Cluster B personality disorders, such as narcissistic personality disorder or borderline personality disorder (Table 6–5). Clinicians should evaluate patients for psychiatric conditions commonly comorbid with CSBD, such as ADHD, anxiety disorders, and depression (Table 6–6). A diagnosis of CSBD precludes hypersexual behavior occurring only during the active or acute stage of another psychiatric disease. However, in practice, anxiety, depression, and SUDs commonly co-occur with CSBD.

Because few universally accepted treatments for CSBD are available, assessment often focuses on other disorders that are amenable to psychiatric treatment. The psychiatric assessment can be of enormous assistance in identifying co-occurring disorders and considering effective and safe treatments for CSBD. Although it is beyond the scope of this chapter to detail treatment options, we want to emphasize that the assessment should be completed with the treatment goal of managing not only sexual compulsivities but also any comorbid traits and illnesses.

Table 6–6.   Mental health problems commonly associated with
compulsive sexual behavior disorder (CSBD)

Anxiety Depression Substance abuse disorder ADHD	Anxiety, depression, and substance abuse can be both fuel for compulsive sexual behavior and a consequence of persistent engagement in compulsive and dysfunctional sexual behaviors.
Paraphilias	Paraphilic behaviors are commonly seen in CSBD, particularly fetishistic behaviors and other less harmful (i.e., *not* pedophilia and *not* sex with nonconsenting partners) paraphilic behaviors.
Sexual disorders such as premature ejaculation and erectile dysfunction Personality traits such as low self-esteem and insecure attachment styles	People who commonly engage in compulsive sexual behavior often have concomitant sexual performance issues in their primary relationships and tend to have interpersonal problems that may make long-lasting relationships more challenging.

Disorders related to CSBD have been associated with affect dysregulation (Samenow 2010), depression and anxiety (Bancroft 2009; Kaplan and Krueger 2010), impulsivity (Miner et al. 2009; Raymond et al. 2003), loneliness (Yoder et al. 2005), low self-worth and insecure attachment styles (Zapf et al. 2008), personal distress (Kafka and Hennen 1999; Kingston and Firestone 2008), risk-taking behaviors such as substance abuse (Kaplan and Krueger 2010), and feelings of self-hatred and shame (Kaplan and Krueger 2010; Reid et al. 2008). Using the Mood and Sexuality Questionnaire in studies of 919 heterosexual men and 662 homosexual men, respectively, two separate studies found that only a minority of the samples reported having greater interest in sexual thoughts or activities when they were depressed or feeling anxiety (Bancroft and Vukadinovic 2004; Bancroft et al. 2003).

Anxiety, depression, ADHD, OCD, and mood disorders often occur concomitantly with CSBD. These disorders may predate the CSBD or may arise from complications in a patient's familial, social, and occupational life that are caused by that person's dysfunctional sexual behaviors. They may arise during the chaos of active symptoms; patients who are predisposed to major mental illness may have new-onset pathology that requires treatment. They may even arise during the course of the treatment. When patients confront their illness during the initial crisis period or confront the damage done to themselves and others through their sexual behaviors, severe mental health challenges may occur, and major psychiatric illnesses may become evident and may require medical treatment.

Possibly co-occuring paraphilias/paraphilic disorders require special attention because they may complicate the entire clinical picture and make diagnosis of CSBD difficult. Evaluators should be familiar with paraphilic disorders and paraphilias and their diagnostic criteria. They must question the patient about paraphilic behaviors that are a threat to public safety and potential sexual crimes and be up-to-date with the laws of their jurisdiction regarding dangerousness to self and others and the psychiatrist's duty to warn.

Medical Testing

Any new-onset psychiatric condition or change in mental status summarily requires a full medical workup, including routine chemistry, hormone testing, and, when there is clinical suspicion, neuroimaging and substance abuse testing. As noted, assessment requires a routine psychiatric assessment, with an emphasis on sexual history (Table 6–7). A physical examination should be done to rule out medical conditions that contribute to the sexual compulsivity or have arisen as a consequence of the CSBD and to assess for sexually transmitted diseases. Standard laboratory testing should rule out common medical problems, with a focus on disorders that may affect sexual desire, arousal, and orgasm. Thyroid disease that may cause anxieties and mood disorders should be considered and assessed. A full assessment should include testing of hormonal functioning, including but not limited to testosterone, estrogen, luteinizing hormone, and prolactin levels. Medical conditions that may result in symptoms of CSBD include polycystic ovarian syndrome with elevated testosterone levels and sex hormone–producing adrenal tumors such as pheochromocytoma. Neuroimaging CT and MRI scans may be indicated to rule out contributory neuroanatomical factors, including neurological conditions such as dementia, particularly frontotemporal dementias; Huntington's disease brain tumors in the ventricular region; and closed or open traumatic head injury that may result in disinhibition and hypersexuality.

Hypersexual states may be iatrogenic. Clinicians must carefully elicit data about medications that may increase dysfunctional sexual behaviors. Antidepressants can energize and create disinhibited, manic, or hypersexual states. Although serotonergic antidepressants are typically associated with sexual inhibition, there have been case reports of per-

Table 6–7.   Assessment protocol

1. Complete psychiatric evaluation with a focus on sexual functioning and detailed present illness history

2. Psychometrics

3. Sexual status examination

4. Physical examination

5. Standard laboratory testing

6. Testing for sexually transmitted diseases and hormonal functioning, including but not limited to testosterone, estrogen, luteinizing hormone, and prolactin levels

7. If clinical suspicion, neuroimaging CT and MRI

8. Rule out substance abuse and iatrogenic causes (medications)

9. Assess for sexual dysfunctions

sons with persistent genital arousal syndrome secondary to their use (Leiblum and Goldmeier 2008).

Medications used to treat depression that increase dopamine in particular, such as bupropion, can increase sexual behavior. Similarly, medications used to treat anxiety, such as the predominantly serotonergic and partly dopaminergic buspirone and the disinhibiting benzodiazepines, can increase desire and arousal. Levodopa medications for Parkinson's disease are known to cause hypersexuality. Increased sexual behavior may arise from the administration of corticosteroids and testosterone replacement therapy. Prescribed or recreational use of ADHD stimulant medications, such as methylphenidate and amphetamine/dextroamphetamine, can cause increases in sexual behaviors. Although erectogenics, such as sildenafil and other phosphodiesterase-5 inhibitors, have a physiological impact on the arousal stage and not the desire or orgasm stage, their use may create a positive feedback loop between desire and arousal and lead the person to pursue unusual and adventurous sexual trysts. Over-the-counter antidepressants (S-adenosyl methionine [SAM-e]), stimulants (e.g., caffeine pills), alkyl nitrites (e.g., poppers), herbals (e.g., *Ginkgo biloba*), and testosterone precursor (e.g., docosahexaenoic acid [DHA]) may increase sexual behavior.

Assessment must include testing for the presence of SUDs. Proper evaluation of SUDs is critical and may include toxicology testing to assess whether illicit substances are causing or exacerbating the CSBD. Hypersexual behaviors are often associated with or a result of stimulant drug misuse/abuse (Weiss et al. 2015); some researchers documented that 69%–80% of female, male, homosexual, or heterosexual individuals with SA showed co-occurring addictions (Carnes 2005; Carnes et al. 2005). Aside from seeking a routine assessment of drugs of abuse, examiners should be particularly careful to assess for the use of recreational drugs that are associated with increased sexual desire, such as cocaine, 3,4-methylenedioxymethamphetamine, and crystal methamphetamine. A reasonable suspicion of alcohol or substance abuse may require collateral data from friends and family, toxicology tests, and hair follicle testing.

Psychometrics

As shown in Table 6–8, sexual compulsivity has been measured with two widely used scales, the Sexual Compulsivity Scale (Kalichman et al. 1994) and the Compulsive Sexual Behavior Inventory (CSBI; Coleman et al. 2001). The CSBI is a 22-item scale developed to screen for CSBD. Items are rated on a 5-point scale, with high scores indicating greater CSBD. It contains two subscales: one for control (indicates difficulty controlling one's sexual behavior) and the other for violence (items about being the victim or perpetrator of sexual violence). Each of these scales focuses on sexual compulsions and the focused and intense need to meet one's sexual needs. They also highlight the inability to control one's thoughts, urges, and behaviors related to sex.

Psychological testing can be very helpful in the assessment. The two main psychometric measures used to assess HD in research are the Hypersexual Disorder Screening Inventory (HDSI; American Psychiatric Association DSM-5 Workgroup on Sexual and Gender Identity Disorders 2010) and the HBI, which is a measure of overall control of sexual thoughts, urges, and behaviors, the consequences of hypersexual behavior, and the use of sex as a coping strategy.

These two measures and the HD criteria assess for the use of sex as a "coping" strategy. For example, one of the subfactors of the HDSI is using sex for coping and asks patients to rate items such as "I have used sexual fantasies and sexual behavior to cope with difficult feelings (for example, worry, sadness, boredom, frustration, guilt, or shame)" and "I have used sexual fantasies and sexual behavior to avoid, put off, or cope with stresses and other difficult problems or responsibilities in my life." The HBI also includes "coping" items, such as "I use sex to forget about the worries of daily life."

The SA measures we have used most commonly (some of which are available at recoveryzone.com) are the Sexual Addiction Screening Test (SAST; Carnes 1989), Sexual Addiction Screening Test–Revised (SAST-R; Carnes et al. 2010), and Sexual Dependence Inventory (SDI). The SAST-R

Table 6–8. Psychometric measures for compulsive sexual behavior, hypersexual disorder, and sexual addiction

Measure	Description	Criteria	Cutoff	Sample items
Compulsive sexual behavior				
Compulsive Sexual Behavior Inventory (Coleman et al. 2001)	22-Item scale with two subscales: Control and Violence	OCD and compulsions with sex behaviors that involve disruption of interpersonal functioning	40 (range 22–110)	Control: "Have you felt unable to control your sexual behavior?" Violence: "In fighting, have you been hit, kicked, punched, slapped, thrown, [choked], restrained, or beaten by your current or most recent partner?"
Sexual Compulsivity Scale (Kalichman et al. 1994)	10-Item scale derived from a self-help guide	Focused and intense need to meet one's sexual needs characterized by a sense of loneliness, low self-esteem, and lack of sexual self-control	24 (range 10–40)	"I sometimes get so horny I could lose control." "I think about sex more than I would like to."

Table 6–8. Psychometric measures for compulsive sexual behavior, hypersexual disorder, and sexual addiction (*continued*)

Measure	Description	Criteria	Cutoff	Sample items
Hypersexual disorder				
Hypersexual Disorder Screening Inventory (American Psychiatric Association DSM-5 Workgroup on Sexual and Gender Identity Disorders 2010)	7-Item scale split into two parts referencing actions of the past 6 months; may be unidimensional or have three factors	Level of sexual fantasies, urges, or behaviors and despair or impairment due to these activities	20 (range 0–28) OR 4 items in A and 1 in B (3 or 4 score)	A: "tried to reduce or control the frequency of sexual fantasies, urges, and behavior but I have not been successful." B: "Frequent and intense sexual fantasies, urges, and behavior have caused significant problems for me in personal, social, work, or other important areas of my life."
Hypersexual Behavior Inventory (Reid et al. 2011)	19-Item scale with three subscales: Control, Coping, and Consequences	Use of sex to cope with stress, inability to stop harmful sexual behavior, and sacrifice of goals to pursue sex	53 (range 19–95)	Control: "I engage in sexual activities that I know I will later regret." Coping: "I use sex to forget about the worries of daily life."

Table 6–8. Psychometric measures for compulsive sexual behavior, hypersexual disorder, and sexual addiction (*continued*)

Measure	Description	Criteria	Cutoff	Sample items
Sexual addiction				
Sexual Addiction Screening Test (Carnes 1989)	25-Item scale consisting of Yes/No questions	Tested on self-admitted sex addicts, meant to separate nonaddicts from possible addicts	13 (range 0–25)	"Do you ever feel bad about your sexual behavior?" "Do you ever think your sexual desire is stronger than you are?"
Sexual Addiction Screening Test–Revised (Carnes et al. 2010)	45-Item scale with five subscales: Preoccupation, Loss of Control, Relationship Disturbance, Affect Disturbance); additional items for specific populations (internet users, women, homosexuals)	Same as Sexual Addiction Screening Test, but revised to work across populations	Core=6 (range depends on population)	Internet: "I spend too much time online for sexual purposes." Women: "I have traded sex for money or gifts."

Source. Bianca Acevedo.

has 20 items measuring the general construct of sexual addiction, plus four subscales measuring preoccupation, loss of control, relationship disturbance, and affective disturbance. Among SA clinicians, a commonly used tool is the SDI, which measures problematic sexual thoughts and behavior and the frequency and nature of specific behaviors (Delmonico et al. 1998).

Mr. A

Mr. A was a hardworking 43-year-old attorney, a good parent and loving husband, a pillar of his community, and, for the most part, extremely ethical. He liked to say that sex for him was like cocaine for an addict. "I've always had a huge sex drive," he explained at his evaluation. Mr. A shared something that he had heard a famously drug-addicted sports figure once say: doing cocaine made him feel like he had boarded a rocket ship that catapulted him into outer space. Get into the spaceship, press a button, and away he would go. There was no turning him back from his mission. That is just what desire did for him. As he described it, once he started on his path, turning on a computer to look for sex sites, he was past the point of no return. It took him into an altered state and propelled him into an alternate universe. He became like a person locked in a spaceship; his mind would not let him out. Instead, desire and sexual fantasy kept him in a trance, intent on his mission.

As someone whose sex drive level had run naturally high since his childhood, Mr. A appeared to be primed for greater sexual interest and arousal for as long as he could recall. This fact was compounded by the circumstances of his upbringing. As a child, he had shared a bedroom with a makeshift wall with his sister, and he used to peek at her as she undressed. Once, she let him come into her side of the room and touch her genitals. Later, as a youth, Mr. A's hypercharged sexual urges did not find a ready outlet among his peers. He was not popular with girls and had virtually no dating experience. By his 20s, Mr. A had developed an interest in voyeurism and boundary-invasion sex. As he had done with his sister, Mr. A became a "peeping Tom" in adulthood, looking into women's changing rooms in clothing stores and strolling down nude beaches to ogle women. At one point, he began sneaking into fashion shows by impersonating a security guard so that he could watch the models undress—something that he later could scarcely believe he had actually done.

What Mr. A loved was thinking about sex with women other than his spouse, shutting the door to his office and fantasizing about a potential affair partner. Even at work, he would wind up masturbating for 3 hours continually. He could get completely lost in fantasy. This circuit, strengthened by the frequency of his habit, would drive him into a frenzy of desire that threatened his reputation and compromised his time. When it was all over, Mr. A felt disgusted with himself for the hours spent lost in fantasy and masturbation, not to mention the risk he placed himself in—potentially compromising his reputation at work,

Table 6–9.   Case study: clinical criteria

Have you repeatedly failed to resist sexual impulses to engage in specific sexual behavior?

Do you have a long-standing desire or a history of unsuccessful efforts to stop, reduce, or control those behaviors?

Have you spent excessive time in obtaining sex, being sexual, or recovering from sexual experiences?

Have you frequently engaged in sexual behavior at times when you were expected to be fulfilling occupational, academic, domestic, or social obligations?

Have you continued your sexual behavior despite knowing it has caused or exacerbated persistent or recurrent social, financial, psychological, or physical problems for you?

Do you need to increase the intensity, frequency, number, or risk of sexual behaviors to achieve the desired effect, or do you experience diminished effect when continuing behaviors at the same level of intensity, frequency, number, or risk?

Have you given up or limited social, occupational, or recreational activities because of your sexual behavior?

Do you become upset, anxious, restless, or irritable if you are unable to engage in sexual behavior?

isolating himself from friends and family, and depleting his sexual desire toward his wife. Mr. A said his pornography use competed with and undermined his relationship with his wife. Stressful circumstances posed perpetual challenges. In the months before this evaluation, Mr. A experienced the death of his brother and problems with his teenage children. The strain made his escapes into pornography and fantasy look even more attractive. "Stress pushes me to act out, and you're asking for yourself to be hardwired differently," he explained.

On assessment, Mr. A had mild anxiety and irritability, but he failed to meet the criteria for a major psychiatric mood or anxiety disorder. He met Kafka's criteria for hypersexuality and the ICD-11 criteria for CSBD. He endorsed 9 of Carnes's 10 clinical criteria for sexual addiction (Table 6–9).

On his SAST-R, which has a clinical threshold of 7 for the diagnosis of sexual addiction, Mr. A received a core score of 15. He endorsed the preoccupation with sexual thoughts, feeling that his sexual behavior was abnormal, feeling badly about his sexual behavior, hurting someone by his sexual behavior, illegal sexual behavior, failing to quit a sexual behavior, hiding sexual behavior from others, feeling degraded because of a sexual behavior, neglecting important parts of life due to spending too much time on sex, feeling that sexual desire is stronger than the self, and using sex to escape problems. On a scale of consequences of his sexual behavior included in the SDI, Mr. A mainly endorsed the category of preoccupation/loss of control, endorsing 8 of 10 (80%) of the items related to this category (Table 6–10). In the types of behaviors associated with compulsive sex, Mr. A mainly said that behaviors around pornography were problematic. He noted that paraphilic voyeurism and covert intrusions, such as "peeping Tom" behavior, had been a problem in previous decades, but no longer. Mr. A noted current nonparaphilic behaviors such as being immersed in fantasy about past and future sexual encounters, spending hours in the intrigue of possible (but never realized) sex with potential partners other than his spouse, and neglecting personal and professional responsibilities when immersed in sexual fantasy.

Table 6–10. Case study: Sexual Dependency Inventory scale of consequences

I have had severe consequences because of my sexual behavior.
I have struggled with depression and it appears related to sexual acting out.
I have been sexually abused as an adult or child.
I use sex as a way to feel better (intoxicating, tension reliever, sleeping aid).
I do sexual things that are dangerous or self-destructive.
I have lied often to conceal my sexual behavior.
Often, I do not like who I am because of my sexual behavior.
My life is in crisis because of sexual problems.
I have had a number of crises in my life because of sex.
I find less pleasure now than before in the same sexual things.
My mood can shift dramatically around sex.
I come from a family that was controlling and rigid about rules.
After my sexual behavior, I often feel sad because I hurt people I love.

Mr. A was assessed for his readiness to change based on current levels of psychological motivation, with items that assess precontemplation (not yet ready to commit to change and unaware of a problem), contemplation (aware a problem exists, but remaining ambivalent about making a change), preparation (prepared for a commitment to change), action (now taking action to change behavior), grief stage (grieving the loss of self-esteem associated with mistakes made), and maintenance (developing a plan to maintain change). Mr. A identified himself in the grief stage and extremely high in the preparation, contemplation, and action items (Prochaska and Norcross 2001).

At the end of 1 year of treatment, Mr. A told his physician, "I feel like a new path has been cut into my brain. I do feel like I am capable of happiness and being a happy human being. Yes, I still have urges and once in a while I slip [meaning that he looks at pornography briefly]. I'm human. I'm not a robot. But I'll never stray from my wife. I feel my relationship with my wife gets stronger every day."

Although Mr. A's clinical course is beyond the scope of this chapter, his positive outcome began with the assessment, in which the examiner adopted a compassionate, nonjudgmental approach in order to solicit a candid history. The development of such a nonjudgmental approach is generally part of the training of clinicians who work regularly in the area of sexual disorders and dysfunctions and is particularly crucial for clinicians who both assess and subsequently treat the same patient and for whom the assessment is an opportunity to establish a therapeutic alliance.

CONCLUSION

As controversy rages over the diagnosis of CSBD and its professional and legal implications, many patients continue to experience the symptoms and consequences of this disorder. Many psychiatrists are at a loss for how to help those who struggle with sexual compulsions. The suffering of our patients may, in fact, be one of the more compelling pieces of evidence that the diagnosis of compulsive sexuality is a real diagnosis, regardless of what we call it or whether we like it. While clinicians, researchers, and experts try to settle on a proper diagnosis of this entity and its management, the struggle with unhealthy and compulsive sexual impulses continues to be a very daunting and sometimes dangerous problem for many patients. Thus, a thorough clinical evaluation of such patients is critical.

REFERENCES

American Psychiatric Association: Diagnostic and Statistical Manual of Mental Disorders, 5th Edition. Arlington, VA, American Psychiatric Association, 2013

American Psychiatric Association DSM-5 Workgroup on Sexual and Gender Identity Disorders: Hypersexual Disorder Screening Inventory. Washington, DC, American Psychiatric Association, 2010. Available at: http://www.dsm5.org/ProposedRevisions/Pages/proposedrevision.aspx?rid=415#. Accessed July 26, 2011.

Bancroft J: Human Sexuality and Its Problems. London, Churchill Livingstone Elsevier, 2009

Bancroft J, Vukadinovic Z: Sexual addiction, sexual compulsivity, sexual impulsivity, or what? Toward a theoretical model. J Sex Res 41:225–234, 2004

Bancroft J, Janssen E, Strong D, et al: The relation between mood and sexuality in heterosexual men. Arch Sex Behav 32:217–230, 2003

Barth RJ, Kinder BN: The mislabeling of sexual impulsivity. J Sex Marital Ther 13(1):15–23, 1987

Bartlik BD, Rosenfeld S, Beaton C: Assessment of sexual functioning: sexual history taking for health care practitioners. Epilepsy Behav 7:15–21, 2013

Birchard T: Sexual addiction and the paraphilias. Sexual Addiction and Compulsivity 18(3):157–187, 2011

Blum K, Oscar-Berman M, Demetrovics Z, et al: Genetic Addiction Risk Score (GARS): molecular neurogenetic evidence for predisposition to reward deficiency syndrome (RDS). Mol Neurobiol 50:765–796, 2014

Carnes P: Contrary to Love: Helping the Sexual Addict. Center City, MN, Hazelden, 1989

Carnes P: Out of the Shadows: Understanding Sexual Addiction. Minneapolis, MN, CompCare Publishers, 1992

Carnes P: Sexual addiction and compulsion: recognition, treatment, and recovery. CNS Spectr 5(10):63–72, 2000

Carnes P: Sexual addiction, in Comprehensive Textbook of Psychiatry. Edited by Sadock S. Philadelphia, PA, Lippincott, Williams & Wilkins, 2005

Carnes P, Schneider JP: Recognition and management of addictive sexual disorders: guide for the primary care clinician. Lippincotts Prim Care Pract 4(3):302–318, 2000

Carnes P, Wilson M: The sexual addiction assessment process, in Clinical Management of Sex Addiction. Edited by Carnes P, Adams KM. New York, Brunner-Routledge, 2002, pp 3–20

Carnes P, Murray RE, Charpentier L: Bargains with chaos: sex addicts and addiction interaction disorder. Sexual Addiction and Compulsivity 12:79–120, 2005

Carnes P, Green B, Carnes S: The same yet different: refocusing the Sexual Addiction Screening Test (SAST) to reflect orientation and gender. Sexual Addiction and Compulsivity 17(1):7–30, 2010

Carnes P, Green BA, Merlo LJ, et al: PATHOS: a brief screening application for assessing sexual addiction. J Addict Med 6(1):29–34, 2012

Chatzittofis A, Arver S, Öberg K, et al: HPA axis dysregulation in men with hypersexual disorder. Psychoneuroendocrinology 63:247, 2016

Coleman E: Is your patient suffering from compulsive sexual behavior? Psychiatr Ann 22(6):320–325, 1992

Coleman E, Miner M, Ohlerking F, Raymond N: Compulsive sexual behavior inventory: a preliminary study of reliability and validity. J Sex Marital Ther 27(4):325–332, 2001

Delmonico DL, Bubenzer DL, West JD: Assessing sexual addiction with the Sexual Dependency Inventory–Revised. Sexual Addiction and Compulsivity 5:179–187, 1998

Goldman D, Oroszi G, Ducci F: The genetics of addictions: uncovering the genes. Nat Rev Genet 6:521–532, 2005

Goodman A: Sexual Addiction: An Integrated Approach. Madison, CT, International Universities Press, 1998

Grant JE, Atmaca M, Fineberg NA, et al: Impulse control disorders and "behavioural addictions" in the ICD-11. World Psychiatry 13(2):125–127, 2014

Kafka MP: A monoamine hypothesis for the pathophysiology of paraphilic disorders. Arch Sex Behav 26(4):343–358, 1997

Kafka MP: The paraphilia-related disorders: a proposal for a unified classification of nonparaphilic hypersexuality disorders. Sexual Addiction and Compulsivity 8:3–4, 227–239, 2001

Kafka MP: Hypersexual disorder: a proposed diagnosis for DSM-V. Arch Sex Behav 39(2):377–400, 2010

Kafka MP: What happened to hypersexual disorder? Arch Sex Behav 43(7):1259–1261, 2014

Kafka MP, Hennen J: The paraphilia-related disorders: an empirical investigation of nonparaphilic hypersexuality disorders in outpatients males. J Sex Marital Ther 25:305–319, 1999

Kalichman SC, Johnson JR, Adair V, et al: Sexual sensation seeking: scale development and predicting AIDS: risk behavior among homosexually active men. J Pers Assess 62(3):385, 1994

Kaplan MS, Krueger RB: Diagnosis, assessment, and treatment of hypersexuality. J Sex Res 47:181–198, 2010

Kingston DA, Firestone P: Problematic hypersexuality: a review of conceptualization and diagnosis. Sexual Addiction and Compulsivity 15(4):284–310, 2008

Klein V, Rettenberger M, Briken P: Self-reported indicators of hypersexuality and its correlates in a female online sample. J Sex Med 11:1974–1981, 2014

Kraus SW, Krueger RB, Briken P, et al: Compulsive sexual behaviour disorder in the ICD-11. World Psychiatry 17(1):109–110, 2018

Kreek MJ, Nielsen DA, Butelman ER, LaForge KS: Genetic influences on impulsivity, risk taking, stress responsivity and vulnerability to drug abuse and addiction. Nat Neurosci 8:1450–1457, 2005

Leiblum SR, Goldmeier D: Persistent genital arousal disorder in women: case reports of association with anti-depressant usage and withdrawal. J Sex Marital Ther 34(2):150–159, 2008

Miner MH, Raymond N, Mueller BA, et al: Preliminary investigation of the impulsive and neuroanatomical characteristics of compulsive sexual behavior. Psychiatr Res 174(2):146–151, 2009

Odlaug BL, Grant JE: Impulse-control disorders in a college sample: results from the self-administered Minnesota Impulse Disorders Interview (MIDI). Prim Care Companion J Clin Psychiatry 12(2), 2010

Peterson L, Taylor D, Roddy R, et al: Tenofovir disoproxil fumarate for prevention of HIV infection in women: a phase 2, double-blind, randomized, placebo-controlled trial. PLOS Clin Trials 2(5):e27, 2007

Prochaska J, Norcross J: Stages of change. Psychotherapy 38(4):443–448, 2001

Raymond NC, Coleman E, Miner MH: Psychiatric comorbidity and compulsive-impulsive traits in compulsive sexual behavior. Compr Psychiatry 44(5):370–380, 2003

Reid GJ, Siu SC, McCrindle BW, et al: Sexual behavior and reproductive concerns among adolescents and young adults with congenital heart disease. Int J Cardiol 125(3):332–338, 2008

Reid RC, Karim R, McCrory E, Carpenter BN: Self-reported differences on measures of executive function and hypersexual behavior in a patient and community sample of men. Int J Neurosci 120:120–127, 2010

Reid RC, Garos S, Carpenter BN: Reliability, validity, and psychometric development of the Hypersexual Behavior Inventory in an outpatient sample of men. Sexual Addiction and Compulsivity 18(1):30–51, 2011

Reid RC, Carpenter BN, Hook JN, et al: Report of findings in a DSM-5 field trial for hypersexual disorder. J Sex Med 9(11):2868–2877, 2012

Riemersma J, Sytsma M: A new generation of sexual addiction. Sexual Addiction and Compulsivity 20(4): 306–322, 2013

Samenow CP: A biopsychosocial model of hypersexual disorder/sexual addiction (editorial). Sexual Addiction and Compulsivity 17(2):69–81, 2010

Walton MT, Cantor JM, Lykins AD: An online assessment of personality, psychological, and sexuality trait variables associated with self-reported hypersexual behavior. Arch Sex Behav 46(3):721–733, 2017

Weiss RD, Potter JS, Griffin ML, et al: Long-term outcomes from the National Drug Abuse Treatment Clinical Trials Network Prescription Opioid Addiction Treatment Study. Drug Alcohol Depend 150:112–119, 2015

World Health Organization: International Classification of Diseases and Related Health Problems, 11th Revision. Geneva, World Health Organization, 2019. Available at: https://icd.who.int/browse11/l-m/en#/http://id.who.int/icd/entity/1630268048. Accessed October 23, 2020.

Yoder VC, Virden TB, Amin K: Internet pornography and loneliness: an association? Sexual Addiction and Compulsivity 12:19–44, 2005

Zapf JL, Greiner J, Carroll J: Attachment styles and male sex addiction. Sexual Addiction and Compulsivity 15:158–175, 2008

CHAPTER 7

Pharmacotherapy for Patients With CSBD

Peer Briken, M.D.
Daniel Turner, M.D., Ph.D.

The core criteria for compulsive sexual behavior disorder (CSBD) describe the interaction between sexual excitation or sexual impulses and the ability to control oneself sexually (inhibition). Without specifically mentioning this in the diagnostic guidelines, this description reflects one of the most important theories of clinical sexual science—the *dual control model* (Bancroft 2008). There are also neurobiological correlates for this model, which are currently the target of many research efforts (see overview in Kühn and Gallinat 2016).

Etiological factors within the umbrella structure of CSBD have been shown to be multifactorial. Thus, before a certain form of treatment is initiated, a disorder model should be developed that attempts to exclude certain causes (e.g., an organic disorder) while making others appear particularly likely (e.g., using sexuality as a coping mechanism against negative emotions). Only in this way can we plan targeted therapeutic procedures. If the psychological burden is, for example, mainly caused by moral-religious attitudes toward masturbation or pornography, one should refrain from diagnosing CSBD, but consultation with a medical health care provider could still be useful. This underlines the importance of a biopsychosocial approach to sexual problems that clarifies social dimensions as well as important comorbidities, especially depressive disorders, anxiety disorders, and personality disorders.

Medication is useful, especially in the initial phase or in the context of risk management, and frequently indicated in three core areas:

- To enhance sexual self-control or to reduce sexual drive
- To treat comorbid psychiatric disorders that have a functionality or connection with CSBD
- To treat a combination of paraphilic disorders with CSBD

Recently, Briken (2020) proposed to use the dual control model as a starting point for an integrative therapeutic approach in CSBD. This model assumes that humans have a biologically anchored and relatively independent balance of excitatory and inhibitory factors that influence sexuality. This can be supplemented by social and psychological factors (e.g., also intra-individual), or the model can be extended. In CSBD—simply speaking—excitatory factors predominate over inhibitory factors. This may be related not only to different constitutive correlates (e.g., genetic) or distal experiences (e.g., psychological neglect or sexual abuse) but also to the presence of certain comorbid disorders. For example, a borderline personality disorder can impair the ability to control oneself; a depressive disorder can be associated with coping with sexual behaviors; and sexual urges can be particularly strong in a paraphilic disorder such as exhibitionism.

PSYCHOPHARMACOLOGY AND TESTOSTERONE-LOWERING MEDICATIONS

Naltrexone

Naltrexone is a competitive opioid antagonist that neutralizes the effects of exogenous and endogenous opioids. Tablets are usually taken once a day (50–150 mg). It has a narrow therapeutic range. As a μ-receptor antagonist, naltrexone reduces impulsive behaviors and therefore may be effective across a wide spectrum of addictions involving both broadly defined behavioral addictions and substance use disorders (Mouaffak et al. 2017). Based on data from six published randomized controlled trials (RCTs) on different behavioral addictions, a meta-analysis by Mouaffak et al. (2017) concluded that naltrexone could be a beneficial treatment for broadly defined behavioral addictions. Several case reports and series have provided evidence that naltrexone also could be helpful for patients with CSBD (Bostwick and Bucci 2008; Camacho et al. 2018; Raymond et al. 2002, 2010; Ryback 2004; Savard et al. 2020), but no RCTs are yet available. Naltrexone is contraindicated in patients with severe liver or kidney disease and patients receiving concomitant opioid analgesics. It also nullifies the desired effects of opioids, for example, when used against pain. In general, opioids should be avoided during treatment; if necessary in an emergency situation, the opioid dose may need to be increased. Common possible adverse effects of naltrexone include abdominal pain, nausea, vomiting, muscle and joint pain, headaches, insomnia, restlessness, nervousness, weakness, and a slight increase in blood pressure. Naltrexone is dose-dependent liver toxic and may increase liver enzymes and cause inflammation of the liver.

The recommended starting naltrexone dosage is 50 mg/day. However, data from case series and reports indicate that naltrexone at high doses (≤150 mg/day) may be of greater effectiveness in some patients. From a clinical perspective, Briken (2020) suggested that naltrexone could be considered especially for patients with CSBD and comorbid substance-related disorders such as alcohol dependence, but no empirical data so far support this suggestion.

Selective Serotonin Reuptake Inhibitors

The increased binding of the neurotransmitter serotonin to the 5-HT$_{2C}$ receptors in the brain and spinal cord that is achieved with selective serotonin reuptake inhibitors (SSRIs) is assumed to lead to a general decrease in sexual desire as well as reduced erectile function and delayed ejaculation (Pfaus 2009). Due to their antidepressive effect and general effect on impulse control, SSRIs have shown to be effective in patients with paraphilic disorders who have pronounced sexual urges or comorbid depressive or sexually compulsive symptoms (Kraus et al. 2006). So far, no differences in effectiveness among the different SSRIs have been found, although comparative studies are rare (Greenberg et al. 1996). Most evidence exists regarding the use of fluoxetine and sertraline, although individual studies are available on the effectiveness of paroxetine, nefazodone, fluvoxamine, and escitalopram (Adi et al. 2002).

The same drugs that have been used in patients with paraphilic disorders have been used in the treatment of CSBD. Kafka (1994) found a significant decrease in the number of orgasms per week in a group of 11 patients treated with sertraline or fluoxetine over a minimum period of 4 weeks (Kafka 1994). In the only RCT to date, a significant decrease in sexual desire and masturbation frequency was found in a group of 28 homosexual and bisexual men with CSBD receiving therapy with citalopram compared with placebo (Wainberg et al. 2006).

The typical maximum doses of each SSRI correspond to those used for OCD and should start with the lowest dose. According to clinical experience, sertraline at an initial dose of 25–50 mg is particularly suitable for the titration process and can be slowly titrated up to 150 mg. With paroxetine, the delay in ejaculation time can lead to a risk that patients will intensify their paraphilic or violent fantasies to reach orgasm. From a clinical perspective, SSRIs can be particularly successful when patients with CSBD use sex to cope with depressive or anxious-depressive symptoms. SSRIs are also helpful in the treatment of comorbid impulsivity, compulsivity, and OCD (Briken and Kafka 2007). In the case of accompanying paraphilic symptoms without a risk of hands-on offense (e.g., exhibitionistic disorder or child pornography abuse in connection with CSBD), the use of an SSRI is often helpful as well.

Cyproterone Acetate

Cyproterone acetate (CPA) is a synthetic testosterone antagonist that binds to the androgen receptors in the testes and in various regions of the brain, thus inhibiting the physiological effect of the body's own testosterone. CPA also reduces gonadotropin-releasing hormone (GnRH) and luteinizing hormone (LH) secretion in the hypothalamus and pituitary gland via a negative feedback mechanism, which leads to a decrease in serum testosterone concentrations. The lowered serum testosterone concentrations ultimately lead to a general decrease in sexual functioning and a decrease in sexual responsiveness (Jordan et al. 2011).

There are four double-blind studies in which it could be shown that CPA leads to a significantly greater decrease in sexual desire, sexual fantasies, and sexual behavior in patients with a paraphilic disorder compared with estrogens or placebo (Bancroft et al. 1974; Bradford and Pawlak 1993; Cooper 1981; Cooper et al. 1992). More recent observational studies have also found a significant decrease in sexual desire and sexual fantasies and behavior in men when treated with CPA (Lippi and van Staden 2017), with the decrease affecting both paraphilic and non-paraphilic sexuality.

Adverse drug reactions occur more frequently with CPA treatment than with SSRIs. These result primarily from the reduced testosterone serum concentrations and range from rather harmless side effects such as hot flushes and pain at the injection site to serious effects such as depression, gynecomastia, thromboembolic events, or liver and kidney dysfunctions (Assumpção et al. 2014). A large proportion of these side effects are reversible when the medication is discontinued. Because of the complex risk/benefit assessment, considerable side effects, and necessary follow-up examinations, CPA should only be prescribed or used by specialists. CPA is mainly used in European countries and Canada for the treatment of paraphilic disorders in sexual offenders (McGrath et al. 2010; Turner and Briken 2018; Turner et al. 2019). Given the risk of meningioma, CPA can be used only when other treatments are deemed inappropriate in some European countries such as France or Germany (Thibaut et al. 2020).

Medroxyprogesterone Acetate

Medroxyprogesterone acetate (MPA; Depo-Provera) is a synthetic gestagen that has mainly progestogenic effects and inhibits the production and secretion of GnRH and LH via the negative feedback mechanism of the hypothalamic-pituitary-gonadal axis. Furthermore, MPA directly reduces testosterone serum concentrations by inducing the enzyme testosterone-α-reductase, which deactivates 5α-dihydrotestosterone, and MPA increases the binding of testosterone to the testosterone hormone-binding globulin, thereby reducing serum concentrations of free testosterone.

MPA is available as an oral medication or an injectable depot solution; the depot preparation is preferred because of its higher bioavailability. Several studies on the effectiveness of MPA have been published; however, nearly all were uncontrolled and were conducted in the 1980s and 1990s. Three older, double-blind studies (Hucker et al. 1988; Kiersch 1990; Wincze et al. 1986) showed a superior efficacy of MPA compared with placebo in reducing paraphilic as well as nonparaphilic sexual urges, fantasies, and behaviors. To our knowledge, the most recent study assessing the usefulness of MPA was a retrospective file study conducted in the United States that compared 79 mainly pedophilic sex offenders treated with MPA and psychotherapy with 196 offenders treated with psychotherapy without MPA (Maletzky et al. 2006). This study showed that MPA was superior in reducing deviant sexual behaviors. MPA is used on a regular basis in sex offenders, mainly in the United States (McGrath et al. 2010; Turner et al. 2019).

Side effects observed during MPA treatment are comparable with those found during CPA treatment and include weight gain, hot flushes, pain at the site of injection, lethargy and depression, gynecomastia, and thromboembolic events, as well as liver and kidney dysfunctions. Again, most side effects are reversible once treatment has been terminated. Because of the complex risk/benefit assessment, considerable side effects, and necessary follow-up examinations, this medication should only be prescribed or used by specialists.

GnRH Agonists

The GnRH agonists (e.g., triptorelin [Salvacyl] and leuprolide [Lupron]) also belong to the class of testosterone-lowering drugs and, by permanently stimulating the GnRH receptors in the pituitary gland, lead to a significant decrease in the sensitivity and number of corresponding receptors. This, in turn, leads to a significant decrease in the secretion of LH from the pituitary gland. As a result, the hypothalamus-pituitary-gonadal axis lacks the stimulus for consecutive testosterone production and secretion in the periphery, ultimately resulting in significantly lowered testosterone serum concentrations (Turner and Briken 2018). When GnRH agonists are prescribed, clinicians should know that the desired effect does not occur for 3–4 weeks after treatment begins. During the first 2 weeks of treatment, serum testosterone concentrations may even increase; thus, a direct testosterone antagonist (e.g., CPA) should be used to supplement GnRH treatment initially to keep this "flare-up" effect as low as possible (Turner and Briken 2018).

Three systematic reviews concluded that GnRH agonists lead to a greater reduction in sexual functioning, fantasies, and behavior compared with SSRIs or CPA in patients with paraphilic disorders (Briken et al. 2003; Lewis et al. 2017; Turner and Briken 2018). In contrast to CPA, treatment with GnRH agonists leads to a complete cessation of paraphilic and nonparaphilic sexuality in the vast majority of patients, which, on the one hand, represents a desired effect but, on the other hand, also significantly limits their use; complete suppression of sexuality is the primary therapeutic goal in only a very small proportion of patients with a high risk of sexual offending (Basdekis-Jozsa et al. 2013). In exceptional cases, the use of testosterone-lowering drugs may also be considered for persons with CSBD who do not fulfill the diagnostic criteria of a paraphilic disorder when their risk of committing a hands-on sexual offense is high. In a group of 127 men convicted of a sexual offense who reported compulsive sexual behavior, a significant reduction in sexual urges as well as in the frequency of masturbation was observed under treatment with SSRIs, CPA, or GnRH agonists (Winder et al. 2018). However, the small number of included men treated with CPA or GnRH agonists prevented a direct comparison of the three different medications (Winder et al. 2018).

The side effect profile of GnRH agonists is comparable with that observed with CPA, but adverse drug effects seem to occur somewhat less frequently than with CPA. The regularly observed decrease in bone density with prolonged use of GnRH agonists requires special attention, because density only partially returns to normal after discontinuation of medication (Turner and Briken 2018). Therefore, bone density measurements should be taken both before and regularly during treatment with GnRH agonists, and appropriate treatment should be initiated if the decrease in density exceeds a certain threshold (Thibaut et al. 2010, 2020). Another problem that affects most patients after a longer period of time is a metabolic syndrome with weight gain, blood pressure changes, and increased risk of developing diabetes mellitus. Finally, permanent fertility problems are a significant risk, and patients should be informed of this risk before treatment is initiated. Because of the GnRH agonists' complex risk/benefit assessment, considerable side effects, and necessary follow-up examinations, they should only be prescribed or used by specialists.

RECOMMENDATIONS FOR THE CLINICAL USE OF DRUGS IN PATIENTS WITH CSBD

To Enhance Sexual Self-Control or Reduce Sexual Drive

In particular, patients with pronounced problems in sexual self-control and a high level of sexual urgency (excitation) may benefit from treatment with an SSRI (e.g., sertraline 50–150 mg; escitalopram 10–15 mg) or naltrexone (50–150 mg) in the first phase of therapy. Medication can be helpful particularly for patients experiencing pronounced social consequences of CSBD, such as problems at work, sexual risk behavior, or a predominant occupation with sexual fantasies and behaviors so that other behaviors are hardly possible anymore.

Psychotherapy should be initiated during this first treatment period, which often lasts 6–12 months. Once patients achieve a certain stability, for many the medication can be reduced slowly and then discontinued. Because of their side effect profile, testosterone-lowering medications should be reserved for patients who are at high risk of hands-on sexual offending due to CSBD. Testosterone withdrawal often leads to marked depression, which in turn is important for sexual counterreactions or dysfunctional coping attempts against depression. This medication should only be prescribed or used by specialists.

To Treat Comorbid Psychiatric Disorders

The treatment of comorbid psychiatric disorders with a CSBD connection usually involves treatment of depressive disorders or symptomatic treatment of depressive symptoms, affect lability, or impulsiveness in the context of personality disorders—especially borderline and narcissistic personality disorders. In the case of comorbid disorders, drug treatment should otherwise follow the appropriate guidelines. Longer-term drug treatment of the frequently present personality disorders is not recommended. In the case of comorbid substance-related disorders, treatment with naltrexone can be useful. In patients with comorbid ADHD, stimulant treatment might be a useful alternative.

Drug treatment should always be accompanied by psychotherapeutic interventions. However, drug treatment and psychotherapy are often the responsibility of different practitioners. This opens up opportunities through the clear separation of responsibilities and roles, but it also creates problems, such as difficulties exchanging information or possible splitting between different physicians or different approaches, that can be counterproductive.

To Treat Comorbid Paraphilic Disorders

Treatment of CSBD in combination with paraphilic disorders should follow the recommendations provided in the current guidelines (Thibaut et al. 2020). These guidelines are based on a risk-adapted approach—that is, the therapy becomes more and more intrusive depending on the urgency of the paraphilic symptoms and the patient's risk of committing a sexual offense (Thibaut et al. 2010, 2020). Paraphilic disorders that usually include no direct physical contact between perpetrator and victim (e.g., exhibitionism, voyeurism) fall into the relatively low-risk category, whereas paraphilic disorders involving a desire to use violence or to penetrate the victim (e.g., pedophilic disorder, coercive sexual sadism disorder) are classified as high risk (Thibaut et al. 2010, 2020). The aim of drug therapy is to reduce paraphilic sexual fantasies and behaviors in low-risk patients while maintaining nonparaphilic sexuality if possible, whereby complete suppression of sexual functioning including nonparaphilic sexuality is tolerated in patients in the high-risk category (Thibaut et al. 2010, 2020). All currently recommended drugs probably do not have a direct influence on the content of paraphilic sexual fantasies but have a purely symptomatic effect on sexual drive and urges.

The therapy of patients with CSBD, paraphilic disorders, and a risk for sexual offending should be delivered by forensic psychiatry and sexual medicine specialists. When considering the duration of therapy and the question of possible dosage reductions or medication discontinuation, risk and benefit must always be weighed very carefully. This requires a lot of experience.

Mr. P

Mr. P, age 32, came to treatment after being caught at work watching pornography. This was the second time he had been caught and the first time he had received a warning. Mr. P had been raised in a prudish family in which sexuality was taboo. He had started masturbating with the onset of puberty at the age of 13 but always associated it with feelings of guilt. Mr. P has also been watching pornography regularly since his youth. Watching it in the evening while masturbating became a kind of ritual. Although Mr. P was always somewhat subdepressive, he had never experienced depressive episodes or other psychiatric disorders in a narrower sense. His family history is significant, however; his father had a recurrent depressive disorder and died from suicide when Mr. P was 14 years old (i.e., during Mr. P's puberty). His mother remained without a new partner, and Mr. P had always felt responsible for her. Retrospectively, he could remember that after his father's death he had a phase of increased pornography consumption with masturbation but also strong feelings of guilt about both his behaviors and the death of his father.

Despite some insecurity about dealing with women, Mr. P had no difficulty in meeting them later in life and had never had any major restrictions in his sexual contacts with them. He had had three longer partnerships with quite satisfying sexual activities. In these relationships, he tried not to watch pornography and not to masturbate because he always felt that doing so was a form of cheating on his partner. For a long time, he did not really have a problem with watching pornography, especially during his most recent partnership, and he was surprised when his most recent partner, separated from him and he learned she had been having an affair with another man for some time. She stated that she had been dissatisfied both in her relationship with Mr. P and in their sexuality. She described sexuality with him as "boring," which hurt him very much. When she left him about half a year earlier, Mr. P became depressive. Suicidal thoughts preoccupied him for several weeks. He felt very lonely and disappointed, especially in the evenings. He hardly felt like going to work anymore, stopped going to sports, and saw friends even less often than before. He started to spend regular evenings at the computer, where he would search for pornographic videos—"the optimal movie"—and stimulate himself for several hours, but often not to ejaculation. Three months ago, he surfed onto pornographic sites at work for the first time and promptly was caught by a colleague who came into his room. He had not done any masturbation.

The threat of losing his job frightened Mr. P. He was depressed, had indeterminate suicidal fantasies, felt a lack of drive and interest, and continued to withdraw socially. After preliminary examinations, Mr. P was diagnosed with a depressive episode and CSBD. He was prescribed sertraline 25 mg, which was later adjusted to 50 mg and then to 75 mg. In the meantime, a possible delay of his ejaculation latency was repeatedly monitored in counseling. Mr. P stabilized affectively after a few weeks, and he gained a lot of self-control through an increase in his awareness. Sertraline was slowly reduced (from 75 mg to 50 mg to 25 mg) and discontinued after 9 months. With the continuation of the now weekly psychotherapy, he remained stable in his sexual and depressive symptoms. In psychotherapy, he and his therapist successfully established a connection between his family's taboo attitude toward sexuality in his adolescence and his feelings of guilt about masturbation and pornography; the possible significance of his father's suicide and the parentification of his relationship with his mother in the development of his feelings of guilt; and the triggering event, the loss of a partner who then characterized the sexuality in their relationship as boring.

CONCLUSION

In a multimodal approach, pharmacotherapy should be considered in the treatment of patients with CSBD. Drug therapy involves a balance of benefits and risks; Table 7–1 proposes an algorithm for the use of drugs in CSBD that has not yet been empirically validated and is strongly oriented toward treatment of paraphilic disorder (Briken et al. 2003; Thibaut et al. 2010, 2020). If the patient has no risk of self-harm or sexual offending, psychotherapy alone is usually sufficiently effective (level 1). From level 2, pharmacotherapy should be seriously considered. Certainly, one must critically weigh whether administering drugs prevents the often necessary discussion of affective symptoms and whether taking a medical drug represents simply changing from one counterproductive coping strategy to another. Ultimately, we are often confronted with patients who are severely burdened or in high-risk situations for whom, after careful risk/benefit assessment, medication should be seriously considered and not omitted, particularly in the initial therapy phase and with certain comorbidities. Psychotherapists who do not work in the medical field should cooperate with medical colleagues in this area. Pharmacotherapy with testosterone-lowering medications, especially to treat a risk of sexual offending (levels 3 and 4), belongs in the hands of specialists trained in forensic psychiatry and sexual medicine.

Table 7–1. Proposed algorithm of pharmacological treatment for CSBD

Level of severity	Treatment
Level 1	
Aim: Support the control of sexual fantasies, compulsions, and behaviors without risk of self-harm or sexual offending	Psychotherapy
Level 2a	
Aim: Support the control of sexual fantasies, compulsions, and behaviors	Psychotherapy
With comorbid depression, anxiety	SSRI: Dosage at same level as prescribed in OCD (e.g., sertraline 50–150 mg)
May be used in mild CSBD with paraphilic disorders with low risk of sexual violence (e.g., exhibitionism disorder with no risk of rape or child abuse)	
No satisfactory results at level 1	
Level 2b	
Aim: Support the control of sexual fantasies, compulsions, and behaviors	Psychotherapy
With comorbid alcohol problems, other "behavioral addictions"	Naltrexone 50–150 mg
No satisfactory results at level 1	
Level 3 (only for specialists trained in forensic psychiatry/sexual medicine)	
Aim: Control severe CSBD symptoms with comorbid paraphilic disorders and a moderate risk of sexual violence and a risk of sexual offending	Psychotherapy
No sexual sadism fantasies and/or behavior (if present: go to level 4)	CPA*: oral, 50–200 mg/day (maximum 300 mg) or IM, 200–400 mg once weekly and then every 2–4 weeks or
For compliant patient; if not compliant use IM formulation or go to level 4	MPA: oral, 50–400 mg/day or IM, 400 mg weekly and then monthly if CPA is not available
If CPA and/or MPA are not available in your country or they are associated with severe side effects, skip level 3 and go to level 4	
No satisfactory results at level 2a/2b	

Table 7–1. Proposed algorithm of pharmacological treatment for CSBD *(continued)*

Level of severity	Treatment
Level 4 (only for specialists trained in forensic psychiatry/sexual medicine)	
Aim: Control severe CSBD symptoms with a risk of sexual offending. Moderately high to high risk of sexual violence and severe paraphilic disorders	Psychotherapy Long-acting GnRH agonists, i.e., triptorelin or leuprolide acetate 3 mg/month or 11.25 mg IM every 3 months
Pedophilic or sexual sadism disorder	
No compliance or no satisfactory results at level 3	

Note. CSBD=compulsive sexual behavior disorder; CPA=cyproterone acetate; GnRH= gonadotropin-releasing hormone; IM=intramuscular; MPA= medroxyprogesterone acetate; SSRI=selective serotonin reuptake inhibitor.
*In some countries (e.g. Germany, France), due to a risk of meningioma, CPA is recommended only in patients with a contraindication to GnRH agonists. Level 3 would therefore not be used in these countries. If a medication with a GnRH agonist not possible and CPA is prescribed despite the meningioma risk, annual information and written consent must be obtained.
Source. Modified for CSBD from Thibaut et al. 2010 and 2020 and Briken et al. 2003.

REFERENCES

Adi Y, Ashcroft D, Browne K, et al: Clinical effectiveness and cost-consequences of selective serotonin reuptake inhibitors in the treatment of sex offenders. Health Technol Assess 6(28):1–66, 2002

Assumpção AA, Garcia FD, Garcia HD, et al: Pharmacologic treatment of paraphilias. Psychiatr Clin North Am 37(2):173–181, 2014

Bancroft J: Sexual behavior that is 'out of control': a theoretical conceptual approach. Psychiatr Clin North Am 31:593–601, 2008

Bancroft J, Tennet G, Loucas K, Cass J: The control of deviant sexual behavior by drugs, 1: behavioural changes following oestrogens and anti-androgens. Br J Psychiatry 586:310–315, 1974

Basdekis-Jozsa R, Turner D, Briken P: Pharmacological treatment of sexual offenders and its legal and ethical aspects, in The Wiley- Blackwell Handbook of Legal and Ethical Aspects of Sex Offender Treatment and Management. Edited by Harrison K, Rainey B. Hoboken, NJ, Wiley, 2013, pp 302–320

Bostwick JM, Bucci JA: Internet sex addiction treated with naltrexone. Mayo Clin Proc 83(2):226–230, 2008

Bradford J, Pawlak A: Double-blind placebo crossover study of cyproterone acetate in the treatment of the paraphilias. Arch Sex Behav 22(5):383–402, 1993

Briken P: An integrated model to assess and treat compulsive sexual behaviour disorder. Nat Rev Urol 17:391–406, 2020

Briken P, Kafka MP: Pharmacological treatments for paraphilic patients and sexual offenders. Curr Opin Psychiatry 20(6):609–613, 2007

Briken P, Hill A, Berner W: Pharmacotherapy of paraphilias with long-acting agonists of luteinizing hormone-releasing hormone: a systematic review. J Clin Psychiatry 64(8):890–897, 2003

Camacho M, Moura AR, Oliveira-Maia AJ: Compulsive sexual behaviors treated with naltrexone monotherapy. Prim Care Companion CNS Disord 20(1), 2018

Cooper AJ: A placebo-controlled trial of the antiandrogen cyproterone acetate in deviant hypersexuality. Compr Psychiatry 22:458–465, 1981

Cooper AJ, Cernovovsky Z, Magnus RV: The long-term use of cyproterone acetate in pedophilia: a case study. J Sex Marital Ther 18(4):292–302, 1992

Greenberg DM, Bradford JMW, Curry S, O'Rourke A: A comparison of treatment of paraphilias with three serotonin reuptake inhibitors: a retrospective study. Bull Am Acad Psychiatry Law 24:525–532, 1996

Hucker S, Langevin R, Bain J: A double blind trial of sex drive reducing medication in pedophiles. Ann Sex Res 1(2):227–242, 1988

Jordan K, Fromberger P, Stolpmann G, Müller JL: The role of testosterone in sexuality and paraphilia: a neurobiological approach. Part I: testosterone and sexuality. J Sex Med 8(11):2993–3007, 2011

Kafka MP: Sertraline pharmacotherapy for paraphilias and paraphilia-related disorders: an open trial. Ann Clin Psychiatry 6:189–195, 1994

Kiersch TA: Treatment of sex offenders with Depo-Provera. J Am Acad Psychiatry Law 18(2):179–187, 1990

Kraus C, Strohm K, Hill A, et al: Selective serotonin reuptake inhibitors (SSRI) in the treatment of paraphilia (in German). Fortschr Neurol Psychiatr 75(6):351–356, 2006

Kühn S, Gallinat J: Neurobiological basis of hypersexuality. Int Rev Neurobiol 129:67–83, 2016

Lewis A, Grubin D, Ross CC, Das M: Gonadotrophin-releasing hormone agonist treatment for sexual offenders: a systematic review. J Psychopharmacol 10:1281–1293, 2017

Lippi G, van Staden PJ: The use of cyproterone acetate in a forensic psychiatric cohort of male sex offenders and its associations with sexual activity and sexual functioning. South Afr J Psychiatry 23(1):1–8, 2017

Maletzky BM, Tolan A, McFarland B: The Oregon Depo-Provera program: a five-year follow-up. Sex Abuse 18(3):303–316, 2006

McGrath RJ, Cumming GF, Burchard BL, et al: Current Practices and Emerging Trends in Sexual Abuser Management: The Safer Society 2009 North American Survey. Brandon, VT, Safer Society Press, 2010

Mouaffak F, Leite C, Hamzaoui S, et al: Naltrexone in the treatment of broadly defined behavioral addictions: a review and meta-analysis of randomized controlled trials. Eur Addict Res 23(4):204–210, 2017

Pfaus JG: Pathways of sexual desire. J Sex Med 6(6):1506–1533, 2009

Raymond NC, Grant JE, Kim SW, Coleman E: Treatment of compulsive sexual behaviour with naltrexone and serotonin reuptake inhibitors: two case studies. Int Clin Psychopharmacol 17(4):201–205, 2002

Raymond NC, Grant JE, Coleman E: Augmentation with naltrexone to treat compulsive sexual behavior: a case series. Ann Clin Psychiatry 22(1):56–62, 2010

Ryback RS: Naltrexone in the treatment of adolescent sexual offenders. J Clin Psychiatry 65(7):982–986, 2004

Savard J, Öberg KG, Chatzittofis A, et al: Naltrexone in compulsive sexual behavior disorder: a feasibility study of twenty men. J Sex Med 17(8):1544–1552, 2020

Thibaut F, De La Barra F, Gordon H, et al: The World Federation of Societies of Biological Psychiatry (WFSBP) guidelines for the biological treatment of paraphilias. World J Biol Psychiatry 11(4):604–655, 2010

Thibaut F, Cosyns P, Fedoroff JP, et al: The World Federation of Societies of Biological Psychiatry: 2020 guidelines for the pharmacological treatment of paraphilic disorders. World J Biol Psychiatry 21(6):412–490, 2020

Turner D, Briken P: Treatment of paraphilic disorders in sexual offenders or men with a risk of sexual offending with luteinizing hormone-releasing hormone agonists: an updated systematic review. J Sex Med 15(1):77–93, 2018

Turner D, Petermann J, Harrison K, et al: Pharmacological treatment of patients with paraphilic disorders and risk of sexual offending: an international perspective. World J Biol Psychiatry 20(8):616–625, 2019

Wainberg ML, Muench F, Morgenstern J, et al: A double-blind study of citalopram versus placebo in the treatment of compulsive sexual behaviors in gay and bisexual men. J Clin Psychiatry 67:1968–1973, 2006

Wincze JP, Bansal S, Malamud M: Effects of medroxyprogesterone acetate on subjective arousal, arousal to erotic stimulation, and nocturnal penile tumescence in male sex offenders. Arch Sex Behav 15(4):293–305, 1986

Winder B, Lievesley R, Elliot H, et al: Evaluation of the use of pharmacological treatment with prisoners experiencing high levels of hypersexual disorder. Journal of Forensic Psychiatry and Psychology 29(1):53–71, 2018

CHAPTER 8

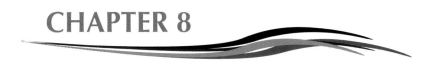

Psychotherapies in the Treatment of CSBD

Rosemary Munns, Psy.D.
Janna Dickenson, Ph.D.
Leonardo Candelario-Perez, Ph.D.
Alex Kovic, Psy.D.
G. Nic Rider, Ph.D.
Dianne Berg, Ph.D.
Eli Coleman, Ph.D.
Abby Girard, Psy.D.

Compulsive sexual behavior disorder (CSBD) is a clinical problem characterized by distressing recurrent sexual urges and behaviors that cause significant levels of distress and functional impairment (Coleman 1992; Coleman et al. 2003, 2018; Miner et al. 2016). This chapter presents an integrative biopsychosocial approach to treating CSBD. We summarize the functions of CSBD, involving the underlying concerns with intimacy formation that contribute to engaging in compulsive sexual behavior. We then describe the modalities of treatment and the tasks accomplished in the course of treatment and illustrate the treatment process using case examples.

In the recent ICD-11, CSBD is defined as a

> persistent pattern of failure to control intense, repetitive sexual impulses or urges resulting in repetitive sexual behaviour. Symptoms may include repetitive sexual activities becoming a central focus of the person's life to the point of neglecting health and personal care or other interests, activities and responsibilities; numerous unsuccessful efforts to significantly reduce repetitive sexual behaviour; and continued repetitive sexual behaviour despite adverse consequences or deriving little or no satisfaction from it. The pattern of failure to control intense, sexual impulses or urges and resulting repetitive sexual behaviour is manifested over an extended period of time (e.g., 6 months or more), and causes marked distress or significant impairment in personal, family, social, educational, occupational or other important areas of functioning. Distress that is entirely related to moral judgments and disapproval about sexual impulses, urges, or behaviours is not sufficient to meet this requirement. (World Health Organization 2019)

Treatment for CSBD focuses on addressing the functions that sexual behaviors serve in a person's life. For this approach, a sex-positive attitude is necessary. Specific types of sexual interests, fantasies, and behaviors are not seen as deviant or nondeviant. *Deviant* is a label used in sex offender treatment to define sexual behaviors that are illegal and that violate the boundaries of others. In contrast, behaviors related to CSBD are based on whether the specific repetitive sexual behavior significantly interferes with the person's social and emotional functioning.

A person's impulsive and compulsive sexual behaviors often evolve over time. Experiences with family and other significant interpersonal relationships affect how a person feels, copes, and behaves. Problems within these relationships contribute to impairment in how the person relates to the world and to him- or herself (e.g., failure to use social supports, lack of interpersonal intimacies, difficulty with assertive communication) (Coleman et al. 2018). Problematic interpersonal relationships contribute to feelings of isolation and disconnectedness and limit the person's access to develop close, rewarding intimate relationships. Often, individuals with CSBD engage in sexual behaviors in an attempt to feel close or intimate with others and believe these behaviors effectively meet their needs. This inaccurate belief perpetuates the behavioral pattern associated with CSBD. The crux of treatment involves challenging the inaccurate belief that intimacy needs are being met and helping patients develop authentic intimacy, with a focus on healthy and positive sexuality (Coleman 1992, 1995, 2011).

Sexual health is a state of physical, mental, and social well-being involving a positive and respectful approach to pleasurable and safe sexual experiences free of coercion and discrimination (World Health Organization 2002). Healthy sexuality involves the ability to have intimate connections with oneself and others, if desired. Identifying, communicating, and living in a way that aligns with one's sexual and personal values, desires, needs, and beliefs is the cornerstone to developing the capacity to form and maintain intimate relationships, if desired (Adams and Robinson 2001; Anderson 2013; Robinson et al. 2002).

TREATMENT MODALITIES

Treatment of CSBD utilizes individual therapy; group therapy; conjoint, couples, or family therapy; partner-specific services; and pharmacological and other medical treatments. Depending on the underlying philosophy of a given treatment program, there are likely to be differences in the modalities used and the ways that they are implemented. However, it can be argued that each of these modalities is important to a comprehensive approach to CSBD treatment, and each should be considered on its own merit.

Treatment may be particularly effective when these modalities work in concert with one another. In order to synchronize treatment with relative ease, the patient sees a primary therapist who also acts as a facilitator of group therapy. This therapist orchestrates conjoint therapy and provides referrals to couples/family therapy, partner-specific services, and psychiatric and medical providers as needed. Exploring the underlying dynamics causing the CSBD is paramount throughout treatment, which requires a careful assessment and an individualized and multifaceted therapeutic approach (Coleman 1991, 2011; Coleman et al. 2018). Thus, we believe that an approach that integrates biological, psychological, and sociosexual theories and concepts is most efficacious.

Individual Therapy

Treatment for CSBD is a principle-based therapy, and we believe it can be employed across most theoretical orientations. In the following, we outline specific tasks that draw from various therapeutic techniques, for example, techniques employed in behavioral therapy for establishing boundaries; traditional or third-wave cognitive therapy techniques that help address maladaptive beliefs about oneself and the world; and family systems, interpersonal therapy, and insight-oriented techniques that help address interpersonal difficulties. Regardless of the specific theoretical orientation of the therapist, building and maintaining therapeutic rapport is essential so that decisions about additional modalities of treatment can be made in the context of a trusting therapeutic relationship. Once other modalities have been implemented, regular individual therapy sessions serve as an anchor to the multimodal treatment process.

Group Therapy

Group therapy is integral to the CSBD treatment process. One of the first tasks of individual therapists is to assess the appropriateness of and patient's goodness of fit for group therapy. This is done by assessing the patient's co-occurring substance abuse, psychopathology, and readiness for treatment and ability to commit to a minimum of 6 months of weekly group therapy. In addition, patients need sufficient social and verbal skills to participate in the process of group therapy, not only to benefit themselves but to be a benefit to others. Participating in a CSBD group addresses isolation, increases accountability for behavior change, provides a safe place to learn and practice emotional intimacy, encourages authenticity, and increases willingness to become vulnerable with others. Group therapy is an effective place to learn and practice these skills under the guidance of the therapists (Coleman et al. 2018).

Often, individuals with CSBD have kept their sexual behavior secret and fear shame with exposure of their behaviors (McBride et al. 2007). As a result, they commonly resist attending a group where they are expected to allow others to know them on a deep level. Thus, although a patient might benefit from group therapy, the individual therapist often needs to address and closely monitor issues of amenability prior to group placement and during the ongoing group process.

Inclusion of Partner and Family in Treatment

Responses to relational dynamics often contribute to the problematic patterns associated with CSBD, indicating a key point of treatment intervention. Systematic incorporation of partners into the treatment process is highly desired. Partners may become involved with treatment in various ways, including conjoint and couples therapy as well as a group experience specifically designed for partners. Diagnostic assessment of the partner is also ideal; significant others may need their own supportive therapy to deal with the consequences of the patients' compulsive sexual behavior and often have their own psychological issues that need to be worked through independently (e.g., Cohn 2014; Tripodi 2006).

Conjoint and Couples Therapy

Conjoint therapy most often involves the patient's partner but may include other significant people in the patient's life. Unlike couples therapy, in which the emphasis is on both people in the relationship and the relational dynamics between them, the focus of conjoint therapy is on the patient's functioning within the relationship. The goals of conjoint therapy are to provide 1) feedback to the patient; 2) observations; 3) a perspective that is often different from the patient's perspective; and 4) a practice ground for the development of interpersonal connectedness and intimacy (Berg et al. 2017). When family members also participate in the conjoint therapy, identifying and addressing negative or traumatic experiences that occurred within the family of origin can be an important goal. If individuals are partnered, incorporating those partners in conjoint therapy early in treatment gives the clear message that the partners are not to blame for the patients' CSBD but can explore and resolve contributing factors as part of the patients' treatment process.

Once the treatment has progressed to the point of addressing how to change their problematic patterns, or cycles, patients become aware of the motivational and contributory aspects of relational dynamics to their cycle. At this phase, conjoint sessions shift to a couples framework (if partnered) in which the focus of the session is on the relational dynamics that *both* the patient and partner bring to the relationship (Cohn 2014). These discussions are critical to establish the foundation from which either conjoint or couples therapy proceeds. Due to the inevitable impact of CSBD on the sexual relationship, one focus of couples sessions also needs to be on exploring sexual health within the relationship.

Partners' Group Therapy

Partners also have the option of participating in a psychoeducational group. In this group, partners are provided with information about CSBD and its treatment, but the group emphasizes general psychological education that can help them cope with their own stress related to their partner's CSBD. Psychological strategies include tools to improve communication, learn ways to set limits, increase social support, and improve their own sexual health. The purpose of bringing together partners in a psychoeducational group experience is fourfold: 1) decrease the sense of isolation and shame partners often experience; 2) provide psychoeducational information designed to empower partners and help them regain a sense of control in their own lives; 3) provide a safe and supportive place for partners to make connections with other partners in order to build their support system; and 4) make decisions about the role they are willing or would like to play in the patient-partner's recovery process. Partners can use the group process and feedback received from other members to focus on changes they want to make for themselves, regardless of the trajectory of their patient-partner's treatment progress.

Additional Modalities

Many patients have co-occurring mental health concerns or a type of sexual dysfunction for which medical treatments involving psychiatry or a physician specializing in sexual medicine may be indicated (e.g., Black et al. 1997; Braun-Harvey and Vigorito 2016; Coleman 2011; Coleman et al. 2003; Raymond et al. 2002). It is important that these issues be identified and addressed as early in treatment as possible; however, they may become more apparent as therapy proceeds. It is also important to rule out, resolve, or manage genetic, hormonal, and neurological or neurocognitive abnormalities or deficits (often with the assistance of pharmacotherapies) (Coleman 2011; Coleman et al. 2018). Thus, having a broad-based referral network in which such modalities can be accessed is key to effective treatment; when used in conjunction with therapy, these modalities prove quite beneficial. Multimodal treatment often involves multiple settings where the patient participates in specific tasks at different stages of the treatment process. This specific sequence of the treatment process and tasks associated with each stage are delineated in the next section.

TREATMENT PROCESS AND TASKS

Initial Phase: Stabilization and Self-Management

The initial phase of treatment helps patients identify and evaluate the sexual behaviors that are causing distress and interfering with their life. Therapists assist patients in putting limits on their distressing behaviors and developing healthy coping skills and resources. Once such behaviors are reasonably controlled, the focus shifts toward understanding the maladaptive patterns that drive these behaviors.

Developing Boundaries

In the initial phases of treatment, one of the first tasks is to enhance the person's ability to develop boundaries. Boundaries are self-imposed parameters set for a behavior the person wishes to change. Using principles of harm reduction (Inciardi and Harrison 2000), boundaries are triaged and prioritized by targeting the most damaging and dangerous behavior first.

Boundaries should not be prescriptive but should be uniquely tailored to the person's context in order to create an experience of gaining control and a sense of agency with the behavior. Many patients who are in the initial stages of treatment have had very little experience with self-agency; they feel at the whim and mercy of their own sexual behaviors. Clinicians must be aware of and comfortable with a wide range of sexual behavior. Without this reflective function, they run the risk of imposing their own values system on patients' sexual behaviors and creating a rupture in the therapeutic alliance. Therapists must avoid reinforcing judgmental and shaming messages regarding sexual preferences. Individually tailored boundaries, free from sexual biases and shame, are consistent with sex-positive and humanistic views of patients as autonomous agents of their own lives.

To identify sexual behaviors ranging from distressing to healthy, patients benefit from completing a comprehensive inventory of their current sexual behaviors. A precise and clear understanding of specific sexual behaviors aids in developing more precise and clear boundaries. Yet when discussing sexual behaviors, many patients use vague, indirect, and figurative language to avoid shame, guilt, or embarrassment about sexuality (Braun-Harvey and Vigorito 2016). Guiding patients to discuss sexual behavior with clarity highlights how these emotional themes can serve as an exposure to shame and other negative emotions. In addition, discussing specific sexual behaviors with clarity prepares patients for engaging in direct communication about their sexual behavior and needs within the context of a group or with their partner(s). Sexual behaviors that should be explored are:

- Engagement in masturbation and other self-stimulation
- Engagement in viewing, collecting, or hoarding sexually explicit material
- Engagement in sexual behaviors with primary partner(s)
- Engagement in behaviors to seek out sexual scenarios, including the use of internet phone applications or websites for dating/cruising; attending bathhouses, sex clubs, or strip shows; and going to bars to cruise or scan for potential sexual partners
- Engagement in behaviors to attract a potential partner, including fixation on unobtainable partner(s), desire to move to another relationship once one has been formed, courtship behaviors
- Engagement in sexual fantasy or sexualization in day-to-day life

Whether in group or individual therapy, once patients list their sexual behaviors, they work to identify whether engaging in such behaviors promotes or impedes their sexual health. Often, they may disagree with their therapeutic team or partners about the degree to which sexual behaviors are problematic (e.g., pornography and masturbation). It is important to identify where patients fall on the spectrum of healthy-to-compulsive behaviors. When a behavior such as masturbation falls into "problematic," this is often due to an internal conflict or a values difference with their partner rather than motivated by compulsion. In these circumstances, couples or family therapy is often recommended to help partners navigate discrepancies.

Many patients have behaviors that they are ambivalent about changing at the beginning of treatment, and using motivational interviewing techniques is vital. Rolling with patient resistance, encouraging discussion about change, addressing ambivalence (Miller and Rollnick 2012), and connecting behavior to values facilitates their motivation to change. Therapists also may engage in techniques of consciousness raising (Prochaska et al. 2006) and mentalizing (Fonagy et al. 2005) about the impact of patients' sexual behaviors on others in their life. This helps them determine whether their sexual practices fit within a healthy or problematic framework.

Involving the partner(s) (if appropriate) in the discussion of identifying and committing to boundaries sets the foundation for providing psychoeducation about sexual desires, fantasies, and interests. It should be clearly communicated and orchestrated that the partner's feedback is not meant for instilling the partner's boundaries on the patient. Rather, the goal is to get the partner's perceptions of the patient's sexual behaviors and to help the patient begin to build awareness of the impact his or her sexual behavior has on others. It is not uncommon for a partner to bring in vital information about the patient's sexual behavior, such as the full extent of the patient's sexualizing of nonsexual scenarios. Once the patient and therapist reach a consensus on sexual boundaries, patients make a commitment to themselves, their partner(s), their therapist, and the therapy group to adhere to these boundaries. Stating intentions for their boundary-specific goals increases the likelihood that they will follow through with those goals (Morewedge and Giblin 2015). Once stability has been achieved and necessary behavioral changes have been established, the deep therapeutic work to address the myriad psychological factors that led them to engage in CSBD can begin.

Understanding Patterns of Behavior and Developing Effective Skills

Although the expectation is to adhere to boundaries, the repetitive and impulsive nature of CSBD renders adherence difficult. Boundary violations offer a learning opportunity for patients to understand their problematic patterns of CSBD and learn better ways of coping with them (Coleman et al. 2018). When boundary violations do occur, patients are guided to explore the topography of the specific sexual behavior and identify antecedents, contributing factors, and consequences of the behaviors while also highlighting necessary points of intervention. This therapeutic task (known as *chain analysis, functional analysis, behavior cycle,* and *behavioral analysis*) assumes that the specific sexual behavior (i.e., boundary violation) serves a function and accomplishes a desired goal, albeit with detrimental consequences (Hayes et al. 1996).

The main steps include identifying an instance of a boundary violation and defining the specific behavior in nonjudgmental and specific terms; collecting information about the context surrounding the behavior (i.e., when, where, and with whom does the specific behavior occur); identifying vulnerability factors (i.e., distal factors that contribute to the behavior, such as quality of sleep, medication use, alcohol or drug abuse, or recent stressful events) and antecedents (i.e., proximal events, trauma, thoughts, emotions that led to the specific behavior); and describing the myriad positive and negative social and emotional consequences of the behavior. Initially, patients often have difficulty determining the precipitating events, believing that their behavior occurs seemingly out of nowhere. Therapists can engage in guided questioning regarding patients' specific behaviors, thoughts, and feelings across a small window of time (i.e., minutes, seconds) that immediately precipitated the decision to break the boundary. Identifying antecedents and the positive and negative consequences of the behavior allows patients to understand the function and effectiveness of that behavior. It is also helpful to explore whether the means of achieving its effectiveness is consistent with patients' values and promotes rather than hinders their sexual health.

Behavior cycles help patients generate insight; allow them to identify links between their behaviors, thoughts, and emotions; and suggest points of intervention from which they can use the coping skills in their current repertoire. This process is conducted over several sessions in which the same behavior occurs, in a variety of contexts, which allows for general themes and points of intervention to emerge. Patients are encouraged to share this cycle with their partner(s) and with their group to enlist their support and to practice honesty and intimacy.

Similar to setting boundaries, we encourage partners to participate (if appropriate) in learning about the patient's behavior cycle (Cohn 2014). Being honest about their boundary violations not only increases patients' ability to be honest with themselves and their significant others but also corrects the negative impacts associated with hiding CSBD. This helps patients build intimacy through sharing emotions and learn to be vulnerable with their partners and other members of their support system.

As patients begin to understand the factors in their cycle that lead toward engagement in a boundary violation, they can begin to build skills to address these vulnerability factors in a process similar to relapse prevention. Every patient will have unique vulnerability factors. However, common factors include negative affect (anxiety, depression, shame); use of cognitive distortions to minimize or rationalize the engagement in a boundary violation; intoxication with substances; and interpersonal conflict. Psychotherapeutic and pharmacological interventions can aid in coping with these factors and may include using medications to manage negative affect; developing distress tolerance to unbearable affects using cognitive-behavioral and dialectical behavior therapy techniques; developing self-soothing abilities when experiencing high negative affect; and developing executive functioning skills, such as stopping to weigh short-term versus long-term impacts and planning ahead for potentially vulnerable events/experiences so that they can put adequate coping measures in place.

Understanding Identity and Addressing Intimacy Concerns

Many individuals with CSBD present with a need to explore their sense of identity and concerns around forming intimate relationships. Thus, to resolve CSBD, concerns related to the self (identity) and others (intimacy) must be understood and addressed. The process of identifying the root causes of such intra- and interpersonal conflicts occurs throughout the treatment process.

Autobiographical History

The goals for the autobiographical history include 1) beginning to understand how the patients' interpretation of life events started to form their beliefs about themselves, others, and their environment; 2) developing insight into how those beliefs influenced their decisions and behavioral patterns over time; 3) developing intimacy and connection with group members and decreasing their sense of isolation as others relate to their formative experiences by saying, "I felt the same as you"; 4) providing a corrective emotional experience through the here-and-now of the group process; and 5) developing an understanding of and taking responsibility for the impact of their behaviors on others. When creating an autobiographical history, patients identify key experiences that have shaped their understanding of themselves and the world. Patients reflect on the meaning and interpretation of past events, experiences, and relationships and how those experiences affected their beliefs about themselves and others. By uncovering the meaning they have made of life experiences, patients are able to focus on underlying psychosocial processes (e.g., attachment insecurity) that have contributed to their beliefs and maladaptive patterns. Patients then develop insight into how these beliefs have influenced their decisions and sexual behavioral patterns. This ultimately helps them understand and take responsibility for the impact their behavioral patterns have had on others. Often, experiences of developmental or situational trauma are identified and focused on at this time. Although the goal is not specifically trauma therapy, dealing with unprocessed or unidentified trauma is key in understanding the aspects of self-and-other that have been impacted in order to better heal and restore healthy processes.

The benefits of the psychosocial history become exponential when patients share these histories in group therapy. By delineating their sexual history, patient become more aware of key events in their psychosexual development, including identity and intimacy concerns. Sharing the key events that shaped their worldview provides an avenue for addressing intimacy dysfunction by creating opportunities for intimacy development. When therapeutically managed, the intimacy and connection built with group members may lead to decreases in shame and isolation, providing a corrective emotional experience (Kell and Mueller 1966). In this way, the potential to experience aspects of authentic intimacy moves toward reality.

For some, sharing their conflicts with family members may be warranted to gain further understanding and a mutual feeling of loss. This process also can be a means of correcting a patient's false narratives that have developed over time. Conflicts within the family of origin ideally are resolved when intimacy functioning in family relationships is improved (Coleman 1995), which is accomplished with family therapy designed to understand the dysfunctional dynamics and develop healthier patterns of relationships. This is true regardless of current relationship status, because many patients with CSBD experience challenges forming and maintaining relationships.

Generalized Life Cycle

The generalized life cycle outlines the general themes developed during the course of treatment. Patients outline the maladaptive patterns that reinforce their CSBD and draw out the generalized life cycle that ultimately led to the CSBD (as well as other problematic behaviors). As they gain coping and intimacy skills, patients also develop a complementary positive cycle. This alternate cycle focuses on healthy coping skills, positive interpersonal interactions, and pathways to engage in a healthy pattern of living. The goal is to help patients develop a healthy view of themselves and their interpersonal interactions.

Developing a Healthy Relationship to Sexuality and Intimacy

Once patients understand their negative and positive cycles, further development of a healthy relationship to sexuality necessitates understanding their erotic interests and sexual values as well as the sociocultural messages that they have internalized (Braun-Harvey and Vigorito 2016; Coleman 2011; Coleman et al. 2018; Money 1980, 1986; Morin 2012). This phase of treatment promotes sexual pleasure in the context of having a newfound sense of stability and control of their sexual behaviors. It focuses on patients exploring and developing a deeper understanding of their sexual interests, fantasies, and behaviors. Such investigation requires a nonjudgmental space in which to explore whether and how their diverse sexual interests fit into their version of a healthy relationship to sexuality. A critical element of this process is identifying patients' personal values and beliefs about sexuality, sexual engagement, and relationships as well as their beliefs about sexuality that have been shaped by sociocultural norms and messages (Coleman et al. 2018). Inter- and intraerotic conflicts often arise between patients' unique erotic interests, their own values system, and the values system of their partners and their sociocultural context. Resolving such conflicts is imperative for achieving sexual health. This therapeutic work centers intimacy, values, and sexual pleasure in their sexual and intimate relationships in adaptive and authentic ways.

As means to exemplify the complexity and work that is done at this stage of treatment, let us look at a brief case example.

Mr. M

Mr. M was a 35-year-old homosexual male with a 10-year history of engaging in compulsive sexual behavior. His behavior manifested in secretly and compulsively searching for anonymous male sexual partners and engaging in receptive anal sex without the use of a condom. He had a partner of 4 years who had stayed with him throughout his treatment process and to whom he was committed and wished to be respectful and faithful. At this stage in treatment, he had gained greater control of his CSBD, but he was now experiencing a sense of loss and confusion about how to go about engaging in fulfilling his sexual life while respecting the

boundaries of his relationship and those he had set for himself throughout treatment.

Through his individual therapy, Mr. M was able to identify that he
erotically was attracted to the idea of anonymity and novelty in sexual
partners. He also recognized that engaging in "barebacking" was more
sexually pleasurable for him than using a condom, and he was excited
by the possible risk of contracting a sexually transmitted infection (STI).
He was also able to identify that although these behaviors excited him
and represented an ultimate form of erotic fulfillment, they did not necessarily align with his values around sex and interpersonal intimacy. Mr.
M valued emotional intimacy and monogamy as well as his own personal health and his partner's health.

Developing a healthier relationship to sexuality involved a process
of individual and conjoint therapy with his partner. Mr. M was encouraged to have an open discussion with his partner in which he negotiated
new boundaries around sex that were fulfilling to him as well as consid-
erate of his partner's values around their shared intimate sexual life.
Both Mr. M and his partner were accepting of having a nonmonogamous
sexual relationship, but Mr. M agreed to not engage in secrecy when it
came to having sex outside of the relationship. Additionally, they were
to "touch base" about their feelings and thoughts about new sexual partners once a month, both agreeing that they did not want to have a poly-
amorous relationship. To address values of physical well-being, Mr. M
and his partner agreed to go on medical pre-exposure prophylactics as a
means to reduce HIV contagion and also to request STI testing from potential new partners. Mr. M came to terms with the idea that complete
anonymity would not be part of his new erotic template and understood
that this shift better aligned his engagement in erotically attractive behaviors with his shared values around sex and relationship intimacy.

As in this case, the ultimate goals of treatment are to develop a positive identity and to build intimacy skills in order to live an integrated
and authentic life. By this point in treatment, patients have achieved a
major transformation in how they view themselves and how they interact with other people, including their partner(s). They also have shifted
how they approach sexual activity with themselves or with their part-
ner(s), resolved any erotic conflicts, and developed positive attitudes
about sexuality.

Maintenance Planning and Aftercare

Living an integrated and authentic life is not easy, particularly for individuals with an extensive history of CSBD. Thus, they may struggle on
their journey. To consolidate the gains they have made in therapy, patients devise a maintenance plan that includes a detailed outline of how
they intend to maintain, consolidate, and continue their growth despite
facing challenges in their life. Patients review their negative and posi-

tive cycles to assist with identifying problematic aspects of their behaviors and engaging in alternate, adaptive patterns.

Patients also actively develop and implement an individualized, positive, sexuality-focused plan for self-care that includes the various tools and skills they have found useful throughout treatment. In creating this plan, patients are encouraged to articulate their boundaries, risks, and triggers and the positive ways they are going to meet their sexual needs for themselves and with partner(s). Patients also identify and make a plan to actively connect with their support system. An important aspect is having patients communicate the role they would like their support persons to play in intervening with negative cycles or patterns and reinforcing positive behaviors. Furthermore, many patients benefit from ongoing psychotherapeutic support to facilitate their journey toward an integrated and authentic life. Such psychotherapeutic support can include an aftercare support group, periodic follow-up appointments, or other formal support systems. Ongoing support helps them maintain their progress and grow further as sexual beings.

CASE EXAMPLES

Mr. O

Mr. O was a cisgender homosexual male in his early 30s who presented to treatment to address difficulty controlling his sexual behaviors after contracting an STI that caused him shame and prompted him to seek help. He presented to therapy in good physical health. During the CSBD assessment, Mr. O described a long history of public sexual activity with strangers, starting with his first sexual experience. Since age 16, he had frequented adult bookstores and bathhouses and often engaged in sexual activity in public spaces. He considered some of these sexual behaviors normative but noted that over the past 6 years, his sexual behavior had become "out of control." Mr. O noted that he spent 2–3 hours a day on various phone applications to seek new sexual partners and engaged in unprotected sex at least four times a week with different sexual partners. He reported that such activity often occurred on the weekend and interfered with his ability to concentrate at work early in the workweek. He also endorsed a history of crystal methamphetamine use. Although he did not believe he had a problem, he acknowledged that each week for the past 6 months he had used methamphetamines at least twice per week while engaging in partnered sexual activity. He reported that his methamphetamine use began 2 years ago and that methamphetamines reduce his anxiety and maximize his sexual pleasure during sexual encounters.

Following the assessment process, Mr. O began to meet regularly with an individual therapist. The therapist provided him with an overview of treatment, oriented him to the treatment goals and process, and clarified the importance of learning self-management and stabilization skills. Mr. O addressed his substance use issues by attending an intensive outpatient treatment program. Individual therapy focused on assessing the types, frequency, and duration of his sexual behaviors. Mr. O oscillated between being overly critical of and minimizing his behavior. He set preliminary boundaries (no unprotected sex with anonymous partners and maintain sobriety from chemicals) but had substantial difficulty maintaining his sexual boundary. It became clear that his emotional dysregulation, particularly related to anxiety, interfered with maintaining sobriety and his sexual boundary. A psychiatric evaluation was recommended, and psychotropic medication was prescribed to treat his anxiety (i.e., sertraline). Mr. O found medication to be helpful in lowering his anxiety, which helped him focus on evaluating his sexual behaviors and adhere to boundaries.

He began tracking all of his sexual behaviors using a chain analysis (see "Understanding Patterns of Behavior and Developing Effective Skills" section). Mr. O learned that his sexual behavior functioned as a way to regulate and manage negative emotions and experiences in his everyday life. He subsequently developed healthy coping skills and found mindfulness and exercise particularly helpful. He also worked on assertive communication to provide him with the skills to discuss safer sex practices.

To facilitate his intimacy-related goals, increase accountability and motivation, and obtain social support, Mr. O began group therapy. Although he initially found the group to be intimidating and struggled with impression management, he nonetheless benefited from hearing others' stories. Once established in the group, Mr. O began sharing his history. He realized he was particularly sensitive to his mother's expectations of him. He needed to be "good" and do as he was told to receive praise and positive attention. He simultaneously learned to hide information to avoid her disapproval and negative interactions. His mother's disapproval, coupled with a lack of sexual education and conversations about sex, fueled his shame about identifying as gay. The feedback process from group and individual therapy led Mr. O to identify the historical antecedents of his generalized negative cycle and his negative core beliefs. For example, his understanding that he had to be dishonest to avoid punishment, in combination with his disposition for anxiety, contributed to the negative core belief of "I cannot mess up." His negative cycle typically stemmed from negative interpersonal events in his life, such as a negative evaluation from a coworker, that would lead to an increase in negative self-talk and emotions. This pattern would intensify when he engaged in compulsive behaviors that he thought would be soothing or numbing. Group therapy provided a reparative experience. He developed trust and intimacy through revealing himself in an honest, vulnerable manner.

Mr. O used his new skills to manage his negative cycle and develop an alternate positive cycle. He sought support from identified people in his life, abstained from using media-based applications, practiced mindfulness, engaged in self-affirming behaviors, and used assertive communication to address points of negative interpersonal conflict in a proactive manner. A positive view of his sexuality emerged with understanding his personal erotic interests and his values around sex as well as recognizing possible areas of dissonance he felt related to sociocultural values around sex. Mr. O completed the tasks and goals of group therapy and moved to a monthly aftercare support group. His monthly group process involved reinforcing his positive changes and living an authentic integrated life.

Mr. H

Mr. H was a 57-year-old cisgender heterosexual male who had been married for 30 years. He presented to therapy in crisis when his wife threatened to divorce him after discovering he had sought services from a sex worker. Mr. H had a history of infidelity (sexual encounters outside the marriage approximately once every other month) and engaged in daily masturbation while watching sexual imagery. He reported that he would sometimes spend 3 hours a day viewing pornography and actively hid these behaviors from his wife (telling her that he was working late). He noted infrequent sexual interaction with his wife. Initially, Mr. H was focused only on saving his marriage and not on changing his behavior. He resisted discussing the details and impact of his sexual behavior.

Mr. H's psychosocial history revealed that he has been raised in the Midwest in a religiously conservative family environment. He was the oldest of three male siblings. He described his deceased father as "good" but distant and cold. He described his mother as "sickly" and his own role in the family as the primary caretaker. Mr. H described himself as a "perfectionist" and was proud of his career and the life he had built for his family. He had two adult children and described his relationship with them as positive, but he focused on their accomplishments and avoided questions related to emotional connectivity. He was self-reliant and denied needing emotional support from others.

The initial individual therapy process was marked by Mr. H's resistance to establishing initial boundaries. He perceived himself as "having it all under control." As such, the first 3 months of therapy focused on addressing ambivalence and connecting his behavior to his goals ("save my marriage"). Eventually, Mr. H committed to deleting all of his pornography and sex-seeking service accounts. He installed a blocking software program on his electronic devices that prevented access to sexually explicit material in order to prove himself to his wife. He successfully maintained these boundaries but noticed that he had a tendency to sexualize women he encountered in his daily life. Mr. H did not want his wife to participate in therapy, and it became evident that he was not communicating with her about his therapeutic process. He felt bothered by his wife asking about therapy, often stating "I don't know what else she wants from me!" The therapist used sexual health principles of honesty, mutual pleasure, and shared values to help Mr. H understand how his behaviors contributed to his relationship distress and were inconsistent with his goal of "saving his marriage."

Conjoint sessions allowed the therapist to gain a different perspective on Mr. H and his relationship. In the initial conjoint session, the therapist helped Mr. H talk to his wife about the principles and goals of the CSBD treatment process. The therapist also discussed the differences between conjoint and family therapy. The therapist helped Mr. H enlist his wife as an ally in his therapy process, with the mutual goal of improving their marriage. During conjoint sessions, Mr. H was encouraged to openly express his confusion about "what she wanted from him." His wife expressed frustration and aggressively demanded, "Let me in." The therapist highlighted the emotions underlying these interactions to increase their empathy for one another. In particular, Mr. H was encouraged to understand and be accountable for how his sexual behaviors affected his wife. Once their emotional expressions softened, the therapist worked with Mr. H to set boundaries about honesty in his relationship. The therapist encouraged him to formulate a plan to increase honesty, communicate about the therapeutic process, and devise a process for being honest with his wife about boundary violations. Because his wife was also ashamed of their current situation and had limited social support, she was referred to a group for partners.

It was clear that Mr. H could benefit from developing intimacy and receiving feedback from others who engaged in similar behaviors. After some deliberation, he agreed to start group therapy. He exhibited difficulty engaging with other group members but was also particularly sensitive about and preoccupied with others' reactions and perceptions of him. Initially, Mr. H became frustrated in group when attempting to share emotionally vulnerable information, and he interpreted the feedback from group members through his core belief lens of "I am not doing it right." Individual therapy augmented the group process by having Mr. H reflect on these group experiences to gain insight about his strong fears of rejection. With this new understanding, he began to talk openly with the group about these fears. The group's empathic response made sharing his history extraordinarily beneficial. By sharing his story, group members validated his difficulty and connected with his experience. Mr. H was able to be vulnerable and tearful in front of other men. He processed shame related to crying, which led to further understanding of how masculine ideals were contributing to inauthenticity. Furthermore, he learned about his tendency to foster closeness with others through his achievements and by providing for others' needs rather than through emotional connection. Over time, he was able to identify his negative beliefs and patterns, all of which revolved around the notion of perfection and avoidance of failure. During group sessions, while focusing on the here-and-now moment, he began to practice emotionally connecting with himself and other members of the group.

Once Mr. H learned how to become emotionally vulnerable in group, he was encouraged to practice doing the same in his marriage. He expressed hesitation, and his fears of rejection and failure became prominent again. At this point, couples therapy was recommended. Couples therapy helped Mr. H and his wife deepen their awareness of relationship patterns that led to repeated disconnection or conflict. They positively shifted their patterns of communication to promote trust building and intimacy.

Mr. H continued to address his CSBD patterns. He identified historical antecedents and negative behavior cycles. He learned that when feelings of inadequacy arose, he sought "sexual release" through sexual imagery or sexual engagement with others. He was able to understand that stressful events in the past few years of his life had left him feeling a sense of loss that he was unable to express and process. This was coupled with an inability to talk to his wife about his own needs. Through an intense process of group, individual, and couples therapy, he was able to build greater comfort with feeling vulnerable and sharing his needs with others, including his wife, when he was feeling inadequate.

After 12 months in group therapy, Mr. H showed confidence in engaging in his positive cycle and reported greater connection with his wife. However, he continued to struggle with reengaging in sexual intimacy with her. In individual therapy, Mr. H was able to explore and process openly about his sexual interests. The therapist worked on increasing Mr. H's comfort with talking about sex in a positive way and normalized his sexual interests. Mr. H learned skills and practiced how to approach a conversation about sex. He was also encouraged to talk about sex in group therapy. With time, he reported increased comfort with his sexuality and that he had reengaged in sexual intimacy with his wife. Through learning skills in group and in his marriage, he developed a positive cycle that emphasized the need to rely on others as well to talk more openly about sex with his wife. At this point, he felt confident in the changes he had made and moved to an aftercare support group. This group provided Mr. H with accountability to his commitments as well as added social support. He and his wife decided to decrease the frequency of their couples therapy sessions slowly over the next year, moving from monthly to every other month. They thought that this was the best way for them to "touch base" with each other as they continued to integrate intimacy, honesty, shared values, and sexual pleasure into their lives.

CONCLUSION

CSBD is a complex and multifaceted problem steeped in interpersonal and intrapsychic distress. Due to the disruption CSBD can cause in all aspects of one's life, treatment calls for an integrative biopsychosocial approach. Although this treatment model reflects current and up-to-date knowledge and practice of CSBD, it has not yet been validated. The goal of treatment is to reconcile concerns regarding identity and intimacy formation by addressing and rewiring maladaptive patterns of responding to stress, emotionality, fear, or distress. We propose that optimizing this integrative treatment approach should include individual, group, and family therapy modalities to honor the complex interrelated systems at play. Therapies involve more traditional behavioral techniques, as well as interpersonal, emotionally focused, and mindfulness-based interventions, that coalesce in a dynamic and multimodal process. By the end of treatment, patients will have established boundaries and intimate relationships that fit into their understanding of healthy sexuality and promote connection.

REFERENCES

Adams KM, Robinson DW: Shame reduction, affect regulation, and sexual boundary development: essential building blocks of sexual addiction treatment. Sexual Addiction and Compulsivity 8(1):23–44, 2001

Anderson RM: Positive sexuality and its impact on overall well-being. Bundesgesundheitsblatt 56:208–214, 2013

Berg D, Munns R, Miner M: Treating sexual offending, in The Wiley Handbook of Sex Therapy. Edited by Peterson ZD. Hoboken, NJ, Wiley, 2017, pp 129–142

Black DW, Kehrberg LL, Flumerfelt DL, Schlosser SS: Characteristics of 36 subjects reporting compulsive sexual behavior. Am J Psychiatry 154(2):243–249, 1997

Braun-Harvey D, Vigorito MA: Treating out of Control Sexual Behavior: Rethinking Sex Addiction. New York, Springer, 2016

Cohn R: Calming the tempest, bridging the gorge: healing in couples ruptured by "sex addiction." Sexual and Relationship Therapy 29(1):76–86, 2014

Coleman E: Compulsive sexual behavior: new concepts and treatments. Journal of Psychology and Human Sexuality 4:37–52, 1991

Coleman E: Is your patient suffering from compulsive sexual behavior? Psychiatr Ann 22(6):320–325, 1992

Coleman E: Treatment of compulsive sexual behavior, in Case Studies in Sex Therapy. Edited by Rosen RC, Leiblum SR. New York, Guilford, 1995, pp 333–349

Coleman E: Impulsive/compulsive sexual behavior: assessment and treatment, in The Oxford Handbook of Impulse Control Disorders. Edited by Grant JE, Potenza MN. New York, Oxford University Press, 2011, pp 375–388

Coleman E, Raymond N, McBean A: Assessment and treatment of compulsive sexual behavior. Minn Med 86(7):42–47, 2003

Coleman E, Dickenson J, Girard A, et al: An integrative biopsychosocial and sex positive model of understanding and treatment of impulsive/compulsive sexual behavior. Sexual Addiction and Compulsivity 25(2–3):125–152, 2018

Fonagy P, Gergley G, Target M, Jurist E: Affect Regulation, Mentalization, and the Development of Self. New York, Other Press, 2005

Hayes SC, Wilson KG, Gifford EV, et al: Experiential avoidance and behavioral disorders: a functional dimensional approach to diagnosis and treatment. J Consult Clin Psychol 64(6):1152–1168, 1996

Inciardi JA, Harrison LD: Harm Reduction: National and International Perspectives. Thousand Oaks, CA, Sage, 2000

Kell BL, Mueller WJ: Impact and Change: A Study of Counseling Relationships. East Norwalk, CT, Appleton-Century-Crofts, 1966

McBride KR, Reece M, Sanders SA: Predicting negative outcomes of sexuality using the Compulsive Sexual Behavior Inventory. International Journal of Sexual Health 19:51–62, 2007

Miller WR, Rollnick S: Motivational Interviewing: Helping People Change. New York, Guilford, 2012

Miner MH, Romine RS, Raymond N, et al: Understanding the personality and behavioral mechanisms defining hypersexuality in men who have sex with men. J Sex Med 13(9):1323–1331, 2016

Money J: Love and Love Sickness. Baltimore, MD, Johns Hopkins University Press, 1980

Money J: Lovemaps: Clinical Concepts of Sexual/Erotic Health and Pathology, Paraphilia, and Gender Transposition of Childhood, Adolescence, and Maturity. New York, Irvington, 1986

Morewedge CK, Giblin CE: Explanations of the endowment effect: an integrative review. Trends Cogn Sci 19(6):339–348, 2015

Morin J: The Erotic Mind: Unlocking the Inner Sources of Passion and Fulfillment. New York, HarperCollins, 2012

Prochaska JO, Norcross JC, DiClemente CC: Changing for Good. New York, Avon Books, 2006

Raymond NC, Grant JE, Kim SW, Coleman E: Treatment of compulsive sexual behaviour with naltrexone and serotonin reuptake inhibitors: two case studies. Int Clin Psychopharmacol 17(4):201–205, 2002

Robinson BBE, Bockting WO, Rosser BRS, et al: The Sexual Health Model: application of a sexological approach to HIV prevention. Health Educ Res 17(1):43–57, 2002

Tripodi C: Long term treatment of partners of sex addicts: a multi-phase approach. Sexual Addiction and Compulsivity 13(2):269–288, 2006

World Health Organization: Defining Sexual Health: Report of a Technical Consultation on Sexual Health. 28–31 January 2002, Geneva. Geneva, World Health Organization, 2002

World Health Organization: International Classification of Diseases and Related Health Problems, 11th Revision. Geneva, World Health Organization, 2019

CHAPTER 9

CSBD in Women

Verena Klein, Ph.D.
Meg S. Kaplan, Ph.D.

Little attention has been paid to compulsive sexual behavior (CSB) in women, who have often been completely absent from research samples. As a possible result, many myths surrounding women's CSB continue to exist. The main focus of this chapter is to review the existing—although minimal—empirical literature on the prevalence, expression, correlates, and assessment of CSB in women. Moreover, the social contexts, such as double standards and gender stereotypes, that interact with sexual behavior in women are critically discussed. Although research on treating CSB is still scant for both women and men and validated therapeutic approaches are lacking, tentative recommendations for psychoeducational and clinical interventions as well as a case example are provided.

Historically, powerful sociocultural forces have curbed the experience and expression of women's sexuality (Meana 2010; Robinson 1984), which resulted in it being seen as pathological and being described using terms such as *frigidity*, *hysteria*, and *nymphomania* (Cryle and Downing 2009). Women's sexual desire has been historically deemed as socially disruptive and problematic (Štulhofer et al. 2016a); for instance, adultery, flirting, and higher sexual desire within marriage challenged the social ideal of the chaste woman and were categorized as nymphomania (Groneman 2001; Tolman and Diamond 2001). In the nineteenth century, nymphomania was first viewed as a medical condition and was treated with interventions such as ovariectomy and clitorectomy before it was reclassified as a mental disorder in the field of psychiatry in the twentieth century (Groneman 2001).

Although recent efforts to integrate the diagnosis of hypersexual disorder (HD) into DSM-5 have failed (American Psychiatric Association 2013), interest in studies on excessive sexual behavior and its nomenclature has increased in the decade since 2010. HD, sexual addiction (SA), or compulsive sexual behavior disorder (CSBD) is characterized as recurrent and intense sexual fantasies, urges, or behaviors that are used to cope with stress or unpleasant mood states and lead to significant negative consequences, such as clinically significant personal distress or impairment in social, occupational, or other important areas of functioning. Individuals seeking help for these behaviors also report unsuccessful attempts to reduce or eliminate their problematic sexual activities (Kafka 2010; Kraus et al. 2018). As with men, CSB in women is characterized by sexual activities such as masturbation, pornography use, and telephone sex (see the section on "Sexual Behaviors" later in this chapter).

Women's sexuality has traditionally been viewed as submissive and less active compared with men's sexuality (Sanchez et al. 2012; Wiederman 2005). In line with this assumption, gender-related stereotypes consider women's sexual desire to be weak and difficult to achieve and men's sexual desire to be spontaneous, strong, and uncontrollable (Attwood et al. 2015; Graham et al. 2017). Study results have shown gender differences in the prevalence of disorders associated with sexual desire that match these gender stereotypes. Whereas women seem to be overrepresented for disorders associated with lower desire (i.e., hypoactive sexual desire disorder), men are overrepresented for disorders associated with higher desire (i.e., CSB; for a review, see Dawson and Chivers 2014). The complicated sociocultural representation of women's sexuality as lacking high sexual desire and levels of sexual behavior (Katz-Wise and Hyde 2014) likely impacts how research has approached the study of CSB. Consequently, little attention has been paid to CSB in women, who were often completely absent in research samples. As a possible result, many myths surrounding women's CSB continue to exist (Ferree 2001); knowledge is based on clinical conjectures and inappropriate generalizations made from research results based on male samples (Montgomery-Graham 2017).

MALE MODEL AS THE STANDARD FOR SEXUAL DESIRE

Criticism has pointed to use of the male model of sexual desire, which does not match with female sexuality. Many studies define *sexual desire* as spontaneous sexual thoughts and fantasies combined with a biological urge and physical changes that result in a need to initiate sexual activity (e.g., masturbation or sexuality with a partner) (Leiblum 2002; Tolman and Diamond 2001; Wood et al. 2006). This model, understanding sexual desire as a spontaneous, biologically determined urge, might lead to the impression that men have more sexual desire than women (Wood et al. 2006). Therefore, it has been claimed that sexual desire is generally conceptualized in line with a male standard of sexuality and does not necessarily match women's sexuality (Kaschak and Tiefer 2014; Leiblum 2002; Tiefer 1991; Wood et al. 2006), and studies have shown that women describe and display sexual desire differently than men (see Brotto 2010). It thus comes as no surprise that sociocultural beliefs determine women's sexual behavior, and a high number of myths about female sexual compulsivity still exist (Ferree 2001). Women who express CSB are even considered "love addicted." The SA literature asserts that high sexual desire that incorporates love and intimacy might be perceived as feminine and that women often are "addicted to" love; men, on the other hand, are often "addicted to" sex. Although the literature emphasizes that women with CSB tend to use sexual behavior as a manipulative instrument in their intimate relationships and to engage in more passive forms of sexual behavior (Turner 2008), this has not been supported by empirical studies (Klein et al. 2014; Montgomery-Graham 2017).

CLINICAL IMPLICATIONS

Traditionally, high sexual desire has been viewed as absent from the stereotype of heterosexual women (Katz-Wise and Hyde 2014); thereby, women who express high sexual desire might fail to adhere to the traditional feminine role. A recent study provided some tentative evidence that mental health professionals are particularly likely to pathologize heterosexual women expressing CSB (Klein et al. 2019). Boundaries between high sexual desire and problematic CSB are not always distinct. Recent research suggests that CSB should not be conflated with involvement in frequent sexual activity and high sexual desire; although CSB is an expression of dysregulated sexuality, high sexual desire in women is associated with positive sexual health and relationship outcomes (Štulhofer et al. 2016b). On the one hand, given cultural expectations, women with high sexual desire might be at risk of being falsely labeled "sexually compulsive" and recommended treatment for problematic sexuality (Štulhofer et al. 2016b); on the other hand, recognizing this disorder in women seems important because "excessively sexually active women could experience increased social stigma and be less likely to express the need for treatment despite pronounced distress from risky sexual behavior" (Öberg et al. 2017, p. e235).

PSYCHOEDUCATION AND CLINICAL INTERVENTIONS

Psychoeducation is an integral part of sexual counseling and therapy. High levels of sexual desire and activity, per se, should not be considered problematic and, in many cases, do not appear to have any particular clinical relevance. Apart from a small subgroup, some women "may be better helped by interventions aimed at reducing self-stigma and internalization of sex-negative norms, as well as by targeting negative consequences in social and occupational functioning, than by focusing on their level of sexual desire" (Štulhofer et al. 2016a, p. 889). Religiosity, which might underlie women's experience of their sexual desire as problematic, should be further addressed as part of psychoeducation.

We do not yet have a clear clinical picture of CSB in women (Montgomery-Graham 2017), and research on treating CSB is still scant for both women and men. Thus far, validated therapeutic approaches are lacking. Hook et al. (2014), in their methodological literature review on the treatment of hypersexual behavior in 14 studies, found that only 4 of the studies had included women in their samples. Cognitive-behavioral approaches were effectively used in two studies. Participants in an online psychoeducational program for hypersexuality (Hardy et al. 2010) reported improvements, but a study that compared cognitive-behavioral therapy (CBT) and art therapy showed significant improvement in both treatment conditions (Wilson 2010). Inpatient therapy (i.e., a 28-day residential program for sexual dependency; Wan et al. 2000) and multimodal experiential group therapy were used to address CSB in both women and men (Klontz et al. 2005). Nevertheless, these study results should be interpreted with caution, because most did not include control groups (Hook et al. 2014).

Although evidence regarding adequate therapy is still lacking, authors have recommended treating CSB with CBT and emotion-focused strategies (Grubbs et al. 2017; Montgomery-Graham 2017). This "comprehensive relational CBT approach" is characterized by cognitive (i.e., addressing dysfunctional thoughts) and behavioral (i.e., reinforcement of more adaptive sexual behaviors) components as well as emotion-focused interventions that address maladaptive coping strategies (e.g., dysphoric mood states). In the past, pharmacological interventions (selective serotonin reuptake inhibitors) have also been used (Hook et al. 2014), but given that those studies did not include women, we are cautious with recommendations. However, in the scant literature we found further recommendations. In clinical practice, it might be worthwhile to include a partner in the therapeutic setting to address relationship issues. In addition, regarding group or self-support groups, those that include women only might be more effective than mixed-gender groups (Montgomery-Graham 2017).

Mrs. B

Mrs. B presented to therapy with the complaint "my sexual behavior is out of control." She was a 30-year-old heterosexual, successful professional woman in a 2-year relationship. She had one child from a previous marriage. Mrs. B was not currently in treatment but had seen a psychiatrist in the past for what she called "emotional dysregulation." She had never been treated with psychotropic medication. She described her current relationship with her boyfriend as excellent but was fearful that her out-of-control sexual behavior would ruin the relationship.

Mrs. B had been brought up in an intact family as an only child. She described her mother as critical and cold and her father as warm and loving but always working. She had no history of sexual or physical abuse. She began masturbation at the age of 9 or 10 and entered puberty at the age of 11. Her first sexual experiences were as an adolescent, where she would have sexual contact with boys in order to be popular. She had married at the age of 24 but was not happy or satisfied in the marriage, sexually and otherwise. She had one child and divorced at the age of 27.

Mrs. B described herself as having had a high sex drive for as long as she could remember. She desired sex more than her partners did and masturbated frequently. However, only recently had it become "a problem" because she felt it was "out of control." She had sexual relations with her boyfriend three or four times a week, which she described as "good" sex. However, for the past several years she would also have sex with strangers she connected with using Tinder, Craigslist, and other online chat and meet forums. She would impulsively do this if she felt lonely. She would go to a man's apartment and have sexual relations, at times not practicing safe sex. Although she knew that this was risky, and she wanted to stop, she could not stop because she found it exciting. She would also have sex with men whom she met in bars. Although she had been doing this for many years and had not ever actually tried to stop, her current relationship was important to her and she did not want to jeopardize it.

She had smoked marijuana for many years and did not consider this problematic. She also had used alcohol since she was a teenager and thought it caused her to be disinhibited sexually and that she drank too much at times. An evaluation by a psychiatrist disclosed that although she was at times "moody," Mrs. B did not meet criteria for manic or depressive episodes. She was advised to see a gynecologist and be tested for venereal diseases and was subsequently diagnosed with chlamydia.

Treatment consisted of supportive psychotherapy and CBT to help her cope with her stressors and emotional problems in a nonjudgmental, sympathetic manner. She was advised to stop drinking alcohol and did this without difficulty. In supportive psychotherapy, she dealt with her triggers, one of which was loneliness, and learned to reach out and communicate more.

Repeated sessions of CBT helped Mrs. B clearly realize that her impulsive sexual behavior was a problem with very negative consequences. She became more motivated to control her behavior and learned to identify its antecedents. Over the course of 1 year she was able to gain control over her unwanted sexual behavior.

In CBT, the emphasis is on the present. According to McGuire et al. (1965), "The theoretical basis for behavior therapy is that the symptom or behavior to be treated has been learned at some time in the past and can be changed by the learning of a new pattern of behavior" (p. 185). CBT interventions have been employed to improve emotional regulation by teaching coping skills to manage thoughts and behaviors as well as identify and change negative cognitions or thoughts. For a more comprehensive review of CBT treatment of the paraphilias, see the article by Kaplan and Krueger (2012).

Mrs. B was motivated for treatment because her impulsive sexual behavior had become a problem and was interfering with her current relationship. This improved with better communication. Other, more general clinical treatment modalities that could be used include mindfulness training (Brotto 2018), helping patients identify healthy sexuality (Irons and Rilke 1994), and dealing with intimacy issues (Schnarch 2009).

CONCLUSION

While we wait for adequate therapy outcome studies, the current state of the art suggests treating CSB using CBT and emotion-focused strategies (Grubbs et al. 2017; Montgomery-Graham 2017). Nonetheless, it is important in clinical practice to consider moral connotations surrounding the presentation of high sexual desire. Particularly in a climate that mixes moralistic, religious, spiritual, self-help, and therapeutic aspects, the risk of false-positives might increase, with serious consequences for targets of counseling or treatment. Recent studies have shown that self-labeling as "sexually compulsive or addictive" correlates strongly with social factors such as shame in a sexually hostile society. This might lead to internalized sex-negative norms and self-stigma and is not necessarily an expression of pathology (Grubbs et al. 2019; Štulhofer et al. 2016b). Thereby, increased awareness of stereotypes and a reflection of one's own gender-role expectations surrounding high sexual desire should be essential in clinical practice. However, clinicians must conduct a thorough evaluation to determine if CSB is present, if treatment is needed, and, if so, what specific treatment is indicated.

REFERENCES

American Psychiatric Association: Diagnostic and Statistical Manual of Mental Disorders, 5th Edition. Arlington, VA, American Psychiatric Association, 2013

Attwood F, Barker MJ, Boynton P, Hancock J: Sense about sex: media, sex advice, education and learning. Sex Educ 15:528–539, 2015

Bancroft J, Vukadinovic Z: Sexual addiction, sexual compulsivity, sexual impulsivity, or what? Toward a theoretical model. J Sex Res 41:225–234, 2004

Baumeister RF, Catanese KR, Vohs KD: Is there a gender difference in strength of sex drive? Theoretical views, conceptual distinctions, and a review of relevant evidence. Personality and Social Psychology Review 5(3):242–273, 2001

Black DW, Kehrberg LLD, Flumerfelt DL, Schlosser SS: Characteristics of 36 subjects reporting compulsive sexual behavior. Am J Psychiatry 154:243–249, 1997

Blumberg ES: The lives and voices of highly sexual women. J Sex Res 40:146–157, 2003

Böthe B, Bartók R, Tóth-Király I, et al: Hypersexuality, gender, and sexual orientation: a large-scale psychometric survey study. Arch Sex Behav 47(8):2265–2276, 2018

Briken P, Habermann N, Berner W, Hill A: Diagnosis and treatment of sexual addiction: a survey among German sex therapists. Sexual Addiction and Compulsivity 14:131–143, 2007

Brotto LA: The DSM diagnostic criteria for hypoactive sexual desire disorder in women. Arch Sex Behav 39:221–239, 2010

Brotto LA: Better Sex Through Mindfulness. How Women Can Cultivate Desire. Vancouver, BC, Canada, Greystone, 2018

Carnes P, O'Hara S: The Women's Sexual Addiction Screening Test. Unpublished measure, Wickenburg, AZ, 2000

Carvalho J, Guerra L, Neves S, Nobre PJ: Psychopathological predictors characterizing sexual compulsivity in a nonclinical sample of women. J Sex Marital Ther 41:467–480, 2015

Chivers ML, Brotto LA: Controversies of women's sexual arousal and desire. Eur Psychol 22(1):5–26, 2017

Conley TD, Ziegler A, Moors AC: Backlash from the bedroom: stigma mediates gender differences in acceptance of casual sex offers. Psychology of Women Quarterly 37:392–407, 2013

Crawford M, Popp D: Sexual double standards: a review and methodological critique of two decades of research. J Sex Res 40:13–26, 2003

Cryle P, Downing L: Feminine sexual pathologies. Journal of the History of Sexuality 18:1–7, 2009

Dawson SJ, Chivers ML: Gender-specificity of solitary and dyadic sexual desire among gynephilic and androphilic women and men. Sex Med 11:980–994, 2014

Dickenson JA, Gleason N, Coleman E, Miner MH: Prevalence of distress associated with difficulty controlling sexual urges, feelings, and behaviors in the United States. JAMA Network Open 1(7):e184468, 2018

Elmquist J, Shorey RC, Anderson S, Stuart GL: Are borderline personality symptoms associated with compulsive sexual behaviors among women in treatment for substance use disorders? An exploratory study. J Clin Psychol 72(10):1077–1087, 2016

Faisandier KM, Taylor JE, Salisbury RM: What does attachment have to do with out-of-control sexual behaviour? NZ J Psychol 40(3):19–29, 2011

Ferree MC: Females and sex addiction: myths and diagnostic implications. Sexual Addiction and Compulsivity 8:287–300, 2001

Gagnon J, Simon W: Sexual Conduct: The Social Origins of Human Sexuality. Chicago, IL, Aldine, 1973

Graham CA, Boynton PM, Gould K: Women's sexual desire: challenging narratives of "dysfunction." Eur Psychol 22:27–38, 2017

Groneman C: Nymphomania: A History. New York, WW Norton, 2001

Grubbs JB, Hook JP, Griffin BJ, et al: Treating hypersexuality, in The Wiley Handbook of Sex Therapy. Edited by Peterson ZD. Maiden, MA, John Wiley and Sons, 2017, pp 115–128

Grubbs JB, Perry SL, Wilt JA, Reid RC: Pornography problems due to moral incongruence: an integrative model with a systematic review and meta-analysis. Arch Sex Behav 48:397–415, 2019

Hardy SA, Ruchty J, Hull TD, Hyde R: A preliminary study of an online psychoeducational program for hypersexuality. Sexual Addiction and Compulsivity 17:247–269, 2010

Hook JN, Reid RC, Penberthy JK, et al: Methodological review of treatments for nonparaphilic hypersexual behavior. J Sex Marital Ther 40:294–308, 2014

Irons R, Rilke RM: Healthy sexuality in recovery. Sexual Addiction and Compulsivity 1(4):322–336, 1994

Kafka MP: Hypersexual disorder: a proposed diagnosis for DSM-V. Arch Sex Behav 39(2):377–400, 2010

Kalichman SC, Rompa D: The Sexual Compulsivity Scale: further development and use with HIV-positive persons. J Pers Assess 76:379–395, 2001

Kaplan MS, Krueger RB: Diagnosis, assessment, and treatment of hypersexuality. J Sex Res 47:181–198, 2010

Kaplan MS, Krueger RB: Cognitive-behavioral treatment of the paraphilias. Isr J Psychiatry Relat Sci 49(4):291–296, 2012

Kaschak E, Tiefer L: A New View of Women's Sexual Problems. Philadelphia, PA, Routledge, 2014

Katz-Wise SL, Hyde JS: Sexuality and gender: the interplay, in APA Handbook of Sexuality and Psychology. Edited by Tolman DL, Diamond LM. Washington, DC, American Psychological Association, 2014, pp 29–62

Klein V, Rettenberger M, Briken P: Self-reported indicators of hypersexuality and its correlates in a female online sample. J Sex Med 11:1974–1981, 2014

Klein V, Imhoff R, Reininger KM, Briken P: Perceptions of sexual script deviation in women and men. Arch Sex Behav 48:631–644, 2018

Klein V, Briken P, Schröder J, Fuss J: Mental health professionals' pathologization of compulsive sexual behavior: does clients' gender and sexual orientation matter? J Abnorm Psychol 128(5):465, 2019

Klontz BT, Garos S, Klontz PT: The effectiveness of brief multimodal experiential therapy in the treatment of sexual addiction. Sexual Addiction and Compulsivity 12:275–294, 2005

Kraus SW, Krueger RB, Briken P, et al: Compulsive sexual behaviour disorder in the ICD-11. World Psychiatry 17(1):109–110, 2018

Laan E, Both S: What makes women experience desire? Feminism and Psychology 18(4):505–514, 2008

Långström N, Hanson RK: High rates of sexual behavior in the general population: correlates and predictors. Arch Sex Behav 35:37–52, 2006

Leiblum SR: Reconsidering gender differences in sexual desire: an update. Sexual and Relationship Therapy 17:57–68, 2002

McBride KR, Reece M, Sanders SA: Using the sexual compulsivity scale to predict outcomes of sexual behavior in young adults. Sexual Addiction and Compulsivity 15:97–115, 2008

McGuire RJ, Carlisle JM, Young BG: Sexual deviations as conditioned behavior: a hypothesis. Behav Res Ther 3:185–190, 1965

Meana M: Elucidating women's (hetero)sexual desire: definitional challenges and content expansion. J Sex Res 47:104–122, 2010

Milnes K: Challenging the sexual double standard: constructing sexual equality narratives as a strategy of resistance. Feminism and Psychology 20:255–259, 2010

Montgomery-Graham S: Out-of-control sexual behavior in women. Curr Sex Health Rep 9:200–206, 2017

Muehlenhard CL, McCoy ML: Double standard/double bind: the sexual double standard and women's communication about sex. Psychology of Women Quarterly 15:447–461, 1991

Öberg KG, Hallberg J, Kaldo V, et al: Hypersexual disorder according to the Hypersexual Disorder Screening Inventory in help-seeking Swedish men and women with self-identified hypersexual behavior. Sex Med 5:e229–e236, 2017

Reid RC, Garos S, Carpenter BN: Reliability, validity, and psychometric development of the Hypersexual Behavior Inventory in an outpatient sample of men. Sexual Addiction and Compulsivity 18(1):30–51, 2011

Reid RC, Carpenter BN, Hook JN, et al: Report of findings in a DSM-5 field trial for hypersexual disorder. J Sex Med 9(11):2868–2877, 2012a

Reid RC, Dhuffar MK, Parhami I, Fong TW: Exploring facets of personality in a patient sample of hypersexual women compared with hypersexual men. J Psychiatr Pract 18:262–268, 2012b

Robinson PM: The historical repression of women's sexuality, in Pleasure and Danger: Exploring Female Sexuality. Edited by Vance CS. Boston, MA, Routledge and Kegan, 1984

Ross CJ: A qualitative study of sexually addicted women. Sexual Addiction and Compulsivity 3:43–53, 1996

Sanchez DT, Fetterolf JC, Rudman LA: Eroticizing inequality in the United States: the consequences and determinants of traditional gender role adherence in intimate relationships. J Sex Res 49:168–183, 2012

Schnarch D: Intimacy and Desire: Awaken the Passion in Your Relationship. New York, Beaufort Books, 2009, pp 1–426

Seegers J: The prevalence of sexual addiction symptoms on the college campus. Sexual Addiction and Compulsivity 10:247–258, 2003

Skegg K, Nada-Raja S, Dickson N, Paul C: Perceived "out of control" sexual behavior in a cohort of young adults from the Dunedin Multidisciplinary Health and Development Study. Arch Sex Behav 39(4):968–978, 2010

Štulhofer A, Bergeron S, Jurin T: Is high sexual desire a risk for women's relationship and sexual well-being? J Sex Res 53:882–891, 2016a

Štulhofer A, Jurin T, Briken P: Is high sexual desire a facet of male hypersexuality? Results from an online study. J Sex Marital Ther 42:665–680, 2016b

Tiefer L: Historical, scientific, clinical and feminist criticisms of "The Human Sexual Response Cycle" model. Annu Rev Sex Res 2:1–23, 1991

Tolman DL, Diamond LM: Desegregating sexuality research: cultural and biological perspectives on gender and desire—ProQuest. Annu Rev Sex Res 12:33–74, 2001

Turner M: Female sexual compulsivity: a new syndrome. Psychiatr Clin North Am 31:713–727, 2008

Wan M, Finlayson R, Rowles A: Sexual dependency treatment outcome study. Sexual Addiction and Compulsivity 7:177–196, 2000

Wiederman MW: The gendered nature of sexual scripts. Family Journal 13:496–502, 2005

Wilson MD: A comparative study of art therapy and cognitive behavioral therapy in the treatment of sexually addictive behaviors and an investigation into the relationship between shame and sexually addicted behaviors in adults. Unpublished doctoral dissertation, Capella University, Minneapolis, MN, 2010

Winters J, Christoff K, Gorzalka BB: Dysregulated sexuality and high sexual desire: distinct constructs? Arch Sex Behav 39:1029–1043, 2010

Wood JM, Koch PB, Mansfield PK: Women's sexual desire: a feminist critique. J Sex Res 43:236–244, 2006

CHAPTER 10

Forensic Aspects of Hypersexuality

Brad D. Booth, M.D., FRCPC
Drew A. Kingston, C.Psych., Ph.D.
Joel Watts, M.D., FRCPC

Sexual preoccupation, compulsion, and addiction and hypersexuality are often used as convergent concepts to describe a high interest in sexual activity that can lead to dysfunction (Brouillette-Alarie et al. 2016). Potential behavioral results include increased sexual partners, higher frequency of intercourse, compulsive masturbation, pornography use, pervasive sexual fantasies, strip-club attendance, and use of prostitutes. In some individuals, hypersexuality may combine with paraphilic interests, with additive problems. Hypersexuality can also contribute to sexual offending.

During the developmental stages of DSM-5 (American Psychiatric Association 2013), Kafka (2010) proposed diagnostic criteria for a new psychiatric disorder, hypersexual disorder (HD). He sought to make hypersexuality a psychiatric illness. Other clinicians made similar proposals for pedohebephilic disorder, hebephilic disorder, and coercive paraphilic disorder. However, experts in the field raised numerous concerns about these diagnoses (Fabian 2011; Fedoroff 2011; First 2014; Frances and First 2011a; Zonana 2011), specifically HD (Halpern 2011; Reid and Kafka 2014). The most serious and most relevant in this chapter was the possibility that the legal system might abuse these diagnoses, thus doing harm to the person or to justice. Normative arousal might be labeled as an illness or might declare a person mentally ill when no illness exists, resulting in stricter or inappropriately lenient sentencing. There is also a lack of consensus about this disorder in the field, resulting in pseudoscience possibly being put forward in court. Socially undesirable sexual behaviors could be inappropriately "medicalized," leading to further stigma of psychiatry and of the sexual behavior. Similar concerns have historically been raised around pathologizing "undesirable" sexual behaviors given the risk of relying heavily on culture and religion to define disease (Davies 1982; Greenland 1983).

Although HD ultimately was not included in DSM-5 (Kafka 2014), the ICD-11 included compulsive sexual behavior disorder (CSBD) as one of the impulse-control disorders (Kraus et al. 2018; World Health Organization 2019). It describes this disorder as a persistent pattern of failure to control intense, repetitive sexual impulses or urges resulting in repetitive sexual behavior. Repetitive sexual activities become the focus of a person's life, to the exclusion of personal care and other interests, activities, and responsibilities. Attempts to control or reduce the behavior fail despite negative consequences, or the person derives little satisfaction from the behavior. The pattern lasts 6 months or longer and causes marked distress or impairment. Distress strictly related to moral judgment or disapproval is insufficient to meet the diagnosis.

As discussed elsewhere (Booth 2016), human sexuality brings an increased risk of legal overlap, including sexual offending. The legal system routinely calls clinicians into legal proceedings as expert witnesses to help fact finders understand why individuals commit inappropriate or illegal sexual acts. Clinicians also educate courts about the risk of future similar behavior and how to manage this risk. Criminal courts are particularly interested in understanding sexual offending. Issues might include sentencing matters, risk assessment, or evaluation for civil commitment under sexually violent predator laws in the United States (Booth and Schmedlen 2006) and dangerous offender laws in Canada. Those who commit sexual offenses could come under the purview of forensic psychiatry if the court finds them not guilty by reason of insanity (NGRI) in the United States or not criminally responsible (NCR) on account of mental disorder in Canada. Forensic clinicians evaluate the role of mental illness in offending and discuss risk management options.

Less frequently, sexual behaviors can come to attention outside of criminal courts, although this could still be conceptualized as a form of sexual offending. Other legal arenas include administrative law, such as licensing of a physician or other professional; family law, such as custody and access issues; and civil law, such as torts, including negligence cases. When entering these legal proceedings, clinicians must have experience working with individuals who have a broad range of sexual and psychiatric issues. They must be aware of the current literature on sexual disorders, such as paraphilic disorders and hypersexuality, and be able to diagnose subtle behavioral presentations of psychiatric and medical illnesses that might mimic CSBD. They need to ensure that they are appropriately diagnosing individuals and providing accurate information within the medicolegal context. In this chapter, we outline important diagnostic issues in hypersexuality that are relevant to medicolegal evaluations and review the forensic and legal issues pertinent to this clinical presentation.

CLINICAL EVALUATION OF HYPERSEXUAL BEHAVIOR IN LEGAL SETTINGS

Human behavior is complex, particularly sexual behavior. When presented with sexual behaviors such as masturbation, viewing pornography, having sexual contact with consenting adults, engaging in cybersex or telephone sex, or attending strip clubs, it important to recognize that such behaviors are not atypical. Similarly, many paraphilic behaviors (e.g., sexual sadism, sexual masochism, fetishism) are common and considered normal in some subcultures (e.g., sexual sadism and masochism in the bondage/discipline, dominance/submission, sadism/masochism [BDSM] subculture). However, these behaviors could escalate to illegal or clearly unethical actions. Regardless of whether considered normal or abnormal, such behaviors could cause dysfunction due to their impact on other areas of individuals' functioning or due to interfering with the rights of others. However, this does not automatically equate to a psychiatric diagnosis or medical pathology—there is a risk of incorrectly pathologizing such behaviors (Halpern 2011).

When attempting to understand complex behaviors, clinicians must employ a legally defensible and systematic approach and be able to present this approach in legal forums such as the court. When doing so for hypersexuality, it is useful to consider inhibiting and disinhibiting factors. These factors could be normal or pathological and may be within (i.e., conscious) or outside (i.e., unconscious) the person's awareness. They could also be a "trait" (i.e., long-standing and relatively stable) or a "state" (i.e., temporary or fluctuating).

> A nursing licensing body has asked you to provide an analysis in the case of a nurse who was discovered to be masturbating to pornography while working nights in the cardiac intensive care unit. She was on her 30-minute break and went to the staff lounge, expecting that the other staff would be occupied on the floor with patient care.

To understand such a case, the clinician must perform a thorough and legally defensible evaluation and develop a biopsychosocial understanding of the person and her behavior (Bradford et al. 2018). Evaluators should first ensure they are qualified to perform the assessment. All available information should be obtained; collateral sources such as family and the workplace should be considered. Evaluees should be warned about the nature of the evaluation, including limits on confidentiality, and understand that the evaluator is not entering a therapeutic relationship with them. Furthermore, evaluees should be made aware that the evaluator's duty is to be honest and independent, which could be helpful, neutral, or harmful to the evaluees' goals. The interview should include typical areas of a mental health assessment, with a focus on sexual issues, disinhibiting factors, and driving factors such as hypersexuality (Table 10–1). Clarification of the sexual behavior is particularly important, including types of behaviors, frequency, conscious motivations, and any resulting dysfunction. One must not equate a sexual incident with psychiatric illness.

Mental health, physical diagnoses, and substance use also require thorough evaluation because they can act to disinhibit individuals or contribute in other ways to sexual behavior. Although testing is not available to diagnose hypersexuality, sexual testing for paraphilic interests, such as phallometric testing or visual reaction time, may be appropriate in some cases. For example, if the case described earlier involved the nurse viewing child pornography at work, then such testing would be recommended. At times, patients presenting with apparently paraphilic behaviors may have a paraphilic disorder that is in part driven by hypersexuality. Alternatively, the paraphilic acts may simply be partly indicative of a broad range of excessive sexual interests rather than a specific paraphilic interest. Unfortunately, no studies have examined this issue. However, our experience is that some people arrested for possession of child pornography do not show preferential arousal to prepubescent children; instead, they show high arousal to numerous paraphilic and

Table 10–1. Driving and disinhibiting factors for hypersexual behaviors

Potential driving factors	Potential disinhibiting factors
Normal wish for sexual outlet/satisfaction	Impaired judgment from alcohol/substances, brain injury, mental disorders (e.g., mania, depression, dementia), intellectual and developmental disorders
Normal sexual drive	
Hypersexual drive, including from compulsive sexual behavior disorder, medications, neurological conditions, and mental illness	Cognitive distortions about behaviors being okay (e.g., antisocial attitudes, dysfunctional processing of own sexual abuse, misplaced ideas of appropriate sexual expression)
Need for intimacy	
Need for happiness	
Escape or distraction from other life problems/self-soothing	Empathy deficits
	Social deficits
Paraphilic interests	Psychosocial stress (e.g., employment, relationships, finances)

nonparaphilic stimuli and describe a high sex drive. As their obsession with pornography increases and they become bored with the materials they have found, they seek out increasingly diverse and sometime illegal images.

Other specialized evaluations also may be needed, such as IQ testing, neuropsychological evaluation, cognitive testing, personality testing, or brain imaging. All of this information could be important to properly understand the behaviors.

PSYCHIATRIC AND MEDICAL MIMICRY IN HYPERSEXUAL BEHAVIOR

To provide expertise around hypersexual behavior, clinicians must be aware of and have experience with clarifying the differential diagnoses for such behavior. Hypersexual behavior can be due to CSBD or be a symptom of psychiatric or medical illness. This differentiation can be particularly difficult for those without sufficient training and experience in the diagnosis and treatment of medical disorders, mental disorders, and sexual issues.

Various physical, mental, and iatrogenic illnesses drive hypersexual behavior. This again highlights the need for thorough assessment by qualified experts.

A lawyer contacts you to request an NGRI assessment of a 62-year-old man with no criminal history. The man is facing two counts of "exposing himself" to strangers. A review of police information reveals that the man lives an apartment building alone and has recently been leaving his door open frequently. Although many have noted his door open, two neighbors saw him masturbating, seemingly unaware of others walking by. He was recently diagnosed with Parkinson's disease and has started aggressive treatment with dopamine agonists. Family confirmed that he has been very forgetful and has been masturbating excessively. He has shown other disinhibited behavior, has pressured speech, and brags that he has the ability to read minds.

In this case, there is a clear overlay of neurological illness with pharmacological therapy as well as some mental health symptoms. An untrained person might assume that exhibitionistic disorder or CSBD is the only problem and ignore the neurological disease and medications as the primary cause of the sexual behavior. Appropriate knowledge of how these issues can contribute is vital so the expert can educate the court.

When acting as an expert evaluator for legal issues involving hypersexuality, one must be aware of the literature on conditions that might mimic hypersexuality and may serve to mitigate or exculpate the behavior. Krueger and Kaplan (2000) discussed neuropsychiatric causes of hypersexuality, highlighting the importance of a thorough history and consultation with family medicine, psychiatry, and neurology. Certain sexual offending populations have increased rates of mental disorders (Booth 2010; Booth and Gulati 2014; Booth and Kingston 2016; Kafka and Prentky 1994), and a portion of these individuals show hypersexual behaviors. Again, appropriate training and consultation are required to recognize and diagnose these disorders.

A summary of psychiatric and neurological illnesses and medications that may induce hypersexual behavior is outlined in Table 10–2 and expanded upon in other chapters.

As an example, courts have examined alternate causes of hypersexual and paraphilic behavior. Devinsky et al. (2010) described a case of a man who developed Klüver-Bucy syndrome, including hypersexuality, after a temporal lobectomy for epilepsy. He was arrested for viewing child pornography. The experts involved were able to recognize that his neurological condition was a significant contributor to his offending, rather than CSBD or a paraphilic disorder. The court considered the Klüver-Bucy diagnosis a mitigating factor. While it may be true that the neurological condition was a primary cause of the offending, some authors have expressed skepticism and have called for caution to ensure that defenses based on behaviors resulting from such conditions are not abused (Steel 2016).

Table 10–2. Psychiatric, neurological, and pharmacological mimics of hypersexuality

Psychiatric disorders
  Mania
  Psychotic disorders
  Depressive disorders
  Autism spectrum
  Substance use disorders and the sequelae
Neurological disorders
  Cerebrovascular disease
  Dementias/neurocognitive disorders
    Frontotemporal dementia
    Alzheimer's dementia
  Multiple sclerosis
  Huntington's disease
  Kleine-Levin syndrome
  Klinefelter's syndrome
  Klüver-Bucy syndrome
  Parkinson's disease
  Seizure disorders and temporal lobe resection
  Traumatic brain injury
Pharmacological/Iatrogenic causes
  Anti-Parkinson's medications/dopamine agonists
  Antipsychotic medications including aripiprazole, paliperidone, risperidone
  Antiseizure medications including lamotrigine
  Antidepressant medications including bupropion, duloxetine, fluoxetine, paroxetine, sertraline, venlafaxine
  Modafinil

Recognizing that hypersexual behavior can stem from other conditions, Kafka (2010) suggested that one should code both the primary condition (e.g., neurological illness) and the HD if the presentation of the sexual issue is chronic. For example, hypersexuality as part of a frontotemporal dementia would be listed as both a neurocognitive disorder and HD. Although coding and diagnosing in this manner has the benefit of highlighting the hypersexual behavior as a special issue in the patient, it could also be misinterpreted as something separate from the underlying cause. Alternatively, it might be labeled "Hypersexual disorder due to another medical condition" to match other DSM-5 conventions; in fact, most psychiatric diagnoses in DSM-5 have exclusions if "better explained" by another disorder. Cantor et al. (2013) also suggested a typology that includes behavior better accounted for by another condition, but the typology was brief, nonmedical, and not looking at psychiatric disorders per se.

STANDARDIZED MEASURES OF HYPERSEXUALITY IN COURT

For evaluating hypersexual behavior, several available tools allow for greater standardization than pure clinical evaluation. A comprehensive assessment should include measure of symptoms and impairment. Although numerous scales are available to help diagnose this clinical presentation, most are not well validated (Hook et al. 2010). It should be remembered that often the condition presents on a spectrum rather than in a dichotomous (i.e., present or absent) manner.

One scale that was developed to examine the negative consequences of hypersexuality, the Hypersexual Behavior Consequences Scale (Reid et al. 2012), shows good psychometric properties. The scale contains two items related to legal difficulties: "I have had legal problems because of my sexual activities" and "I have been arrested because of my sexual activities." In a validation sample of 137 hypersexual individuals, nearly one-fifth had legal problems that they attributed to their hypersexuality, including approximately 10% who had been arrested for nonparaphilic sexual activities such as soliciting sex from a prostitute.

In the forensic arena, experts must be knowledgeable in the measurement and diagnosis of hypersexuality and CSBD. Although literature around hypersexuality and CSBD is growing, controversy also exists, and a court might consider the field to be novel science. Special legal issues relating to novel science and court standards are discussed later in this chapter. When putting these areas into the court, experts must present a balanced view, including highlighting areas of weaker science and of controversy. At times, standardized scales may give the court a false impression of increased validity or acceptance of the diagnosis that experts must clarify.

CURRENT ROLE OF HYPERSEXUALITY IN U.S. AND CANADIAN COURTS

Ley et al. (2015) searched the legal literature back to 1990 examining the prevalence of sexual addiction (SA) being used in U.S. case law. Although this was not an exhaustive search, they identified 210 cases in different branches of law, including administrative (i.e., rules and regulations governing the licensing of professionals), civil (i.e., cases between parties, including suing for damages), family (i.e., child custody and divorce proceedings), and criminal (i.e., violations of law resulting in penalty from governing bodies).

Administrative law cases included both physicians and lawyers who had breached professional standards and raised SA as a mitigating factor. Licensing bodies appeared varied in their consideration of these defenses. Some would accept this as an issue and mandate treatment for SA as part of ongoing monitoring and board-sanctioned assistance.

In civil law, diverse suits arise that use SA as an issue. Most relevant appears to be when individuals are incorrectly labeled as "sex addicts" by a professional such as a psychologist or psychiatrist. Thus, the professional could be liable for damage to a plaintiff. There have also been unsuccessful complaints that SA was not treated appropriately for prisoners and, in another unsuccessful case, that the disorder was caused and fueled by computer companies.

In family law matters, SA has rarely been raised, but when it does appear, it is most often raised by one spouse against the other, usually to present the person in a negative light. This allegation has received variable acceptance by the courts.

Finally, SA is raised most often in criminal law matters. This includes the intersection with civil law in the United States wherein sexual offenders can be civilly committed due to potential risk. Thus, SA may be raised by defense lawyers as a mitigating factor for serious sentences or by prosecutors as an aggravating factor to paint the offender in a negative light.

In an analysis in 2017, Montgomery-Graham searched a large Canadian legal database dating back to the 1800s for cases involving the search terms *sex addiction, compulsive sexual behavior,* and *hypersexual.* This yielded 111 cases plus another 3 referenced cases. Only 48 cases had enough content for review. Interestingly, of the 66 cases not analyzed, 47 were under the criminal review board for those found NCR, and 6 were under a provincial tribunal evaluating capacity to consent to treatment and involuntary hospitalization. This group also included most of the cases found using the search term *hypersexual* (53 of 76 cases).

Cases in the Montgomery-Graham (2017) series fell into domains similar to those in U.S. case law. Administrative law cases (9 of 48) involved professionals who had breached professional standards and raised hypersexuality as a mitigating factor. This had variable impact, although tribunals focused on actual behaviors and risk rather than on the presence of hypersexuality. In one case, there was an enduring pattern of inappropriate behavior and, in another case, a long period of stability and apparent remission of inappropriate behavior. This Canadian study revealed a unique immigration case in which an American reported that he was a "sex addict" with a substance use disorder. His deportation order from Canada was stayed because he would not get access to the same treatment in the United States for his "addictions."

No civil law cases were highlighted, but nine family law cases were noted. Most involved women raising concerns about their ex-spouses being sexual addicts, suggesting that this should be an issue in custody. The author noted that this was not successful because the women presented as "angry, theatrical, or mentally unwell, and awarding custody to these particular mothers would not have been in the best interests of their children" (Montgomery-Graham 2017, p. 210). In one case, a father temporarily lost custody for SA until assessed by a psychiatrist.

Like the U.S. cases, most Canadian cases were in criminal law (30 of 48) (Montgomery-Graham 2017). These cases are not discussed in detail, but the author noted that most involved hypersexuality being raised as a mitigating factor in sentencing. Concern was noted that attendance at a 12-step program for SA appeared to be accepted as a mitigating factor despite the paucity of evidence to support this as a risk reduction strategy in sexual offending.

POTENTIAL APPLICATIONS OF HYPERSEXUALITY IN THE LEGAL REALM

Although hypersexuality has already migrated into all legal branches of jurisprudence in U.S. and Canadian courts, forensic experts must evaluate these issues thoroughly and ensure legal decision makers are appropriately and accurately educated. We discuss potential issues important for the courts in the subsections that follow.

Not Guilty by Reason of Insanity and Not Criminally Responsible Defenses

NGRI and NCR are affirmative legal defenses available in most U.S. jurisdictions and in Canada, respectively. They allow for mental illness that impairs a person's knowledge of wrongfulness to act as a defense to avoid punishment for the crime. However, these defenses are rarely employed for sexual offenses. For example, only about 10% of a large forensic hospital cross-sectional population (Novak et al. 2007) had sexual offenses for which they were found NCR/NGRI. This is partly because there is often a "rational motive" for the behavior, even in those with severe mental illness. Thus even defendants with active psychosis can be found responsible for sexual offenses, although their illness may be a mitigating factor in sentencing.

Similarly, it is unlikely that a person motivated in part by CSBD or hypersexuality from other causes would meet the criteria for most NCR or NGRI jurisdictions. The usual requirement is that due to mental disorder, the person was unable to understand the nature and quality or the wrongfulness/criminality of the act. In some jurisdictions, individuals maybe be found NGRI due to an "irresistible impulse." This is also called the "police officer at the elbow test"—in other words, although the person knew the behavior was wrong, he or she was disinhibited to such a degree that the person would have done the activity even if there were a police officer present. An example might be a patient with bipolar disorder who assaults someone while in the thrall of mania. It would be unlikely a person would meet any of these statutes due to a pure HD.

Some individuals may have underlying diagnoses from which their hypersexual or other sexual behavior stems. For example, a person with undiagnosed frontotemporal dementia may be unable to recognize that the sexual behavior is wrong, thus possibly opening up a legal defense.

Mitigating Factors

Mitigating factors are issues considered by the court that, although they do not exculpate a person, may lessen that person's responsibility and therefore lessen the punishment. Thus, having a diagnosis of CSBD or hypersexuality from other causes could be presented as an illness contributing to the behavior. As noted by both Ley et al. (2015) and Montgomery-Graham (2017), CSBD and hypersexuality diagnoses have been put forward in various cases as mitigating factors. It has long been held in law that a variety of factors can be taken into consideration during sentencing. Although evidence suggests that induced states of hypersexuality are possible, research indicates that hypersexual states can be induced by changes in the frontal lobe, amygdala, hippocampus, hypothalamus, and reward-processing areas of the brain in addition to the dopamine system (Kühn and Gallinat 2016). These intrinsic variations might again suggest pathology, which could be argued to make one less culpable and therefore deserving of a lesser degree of punishment, but this is often left to judicial discretion.

Setting aside the controversies about the validity of the CSBD diagnosis, several other issues are important to note:

- The court, not medical experts, decides the meaning of legal terms of art. For example, although clinicians use DSM to define a mental disorder, such as antisocial personality disorder, the court decides if the diagnosis is relevant or if qualified diagnoses apply to certain legislation. Thus, although *we* may define hypersexuality as a disorder, the court may not, and vice versa.

- Although a mental disorder may have contributed significantly to a person's behavior, multiple factors are often involved. For example, a person may have CSBD and been arrested multiple times for solicitation of prostitutes. However, that person may also have other factors not related to mental illness, such as being single and lonely, having distorted cognitions about the status of women as "objects," and having a high income that makes such activities financially "easy." It is important to highlight relevant contributing factors while realizing that the court will decide their importance for sentencing.
- As with other mental health issues, when examining hypersexuality, the court may also be interested in whether individuals have insight into their difficulties, whether they are making efforts to seek treatment, and whether they have obtained some stability. All these questions may be relevant for appreciating the risk they pose of similar behavior in the future.

Aggravating Factors

Aggravating factors are issues considered by the court that increase culpability because they make an offense more reprehensible. For example, a sexual crime against a pregnant woman might be considered worse than a similar offense against a nonpregnant woman. While CSBD may serve to reduce culpability for some individuals, it may serve to worsen things for others. For example, repeat offending is often considered an aggravating factor by the legal system. It is foreseeable that a person driven in part by hypersexuality would have more than one offense or victim. Furthermore, that person may not have demonstrated any treatment response, suggesting to the court that he or she poses an increased risk. As noted, this issue has arisen in some family court circumstances wherein one spouse suggests that the other, afflicted spouse poses a risk to their child or is an inappropriate parent given their sexual disorder.

This may be particularly relevant in situations in which risk assessment is paramount. For example, in the United States, sexually violent predator laws allow for civil commitment of individuals with sexual offenses (Booth and Schmedlen 2006). Often, these laws will identify that the person has a mental condition. It is foreseeable that CSBD could qualify, forming the basis of the civil commitment. Similar concerns have been raised about paraphilic disorder diagnoses being used in these contexts, particularly when there is controversy in the literature about their validity (Fabian 2011; First and Halon 2008; Frances and First 2011b; Frances and Wollert 2012).

Similarly, Canada has dangerous offender and long-term offender designations that can be imposed at sentencing, particularly in individuals with sexual offenses. This allows for indefinite sentencing and long-term community supervision with intensive oversight. The legislation requires that individuals pose a future risk due to their inability to restrain their behavior. It could be argued that, in some individuals, hypersexuality adds to such a risk; as we discuss in the next section, this issue should be considered in risk assessment.

Risk Assessment

When giving an expert opinion about the risk posed by a person with inappropriate sexual behavior, one must consider all relevant issues of risk. As noted, an important first step is completing an appropriate evaluation, including looking for relevant medical, psychiatric, and medication issues that may explain the behavior. This will form part of the opinion on risk. In addition, hypersexuality may also be relevant.

Currently, the literature shows mixed evidence about the role of hypersexuality in contributing to sexual recidivism. Formal diagnostic criteria for CSBD and HD have not been used in the development of any risk assessment tools; instead, some studies have looked at various indicators that may overlap with these constructs. Thus, the role of CSBD and HD on offending remains unknown.

In an analysis by Etzler et al. (2018) of the predictive capacity of the Stable-2007, which measures enduring but possibly changeable factors, factor analysis confirmed that what the authors termed "hypersexuality" was one of three different factors in the instrument, in addition to antisociality and sexual deviance, and included sex drive/preoccupation and sex as coping measures. Antisociality predicted general and nonsexual violent recidivism and, to a lesser extent, sexual recidivism. Sexual deviance predicted increased sexual reoffending and decreased risk of general and nonsexual violent offenses. Hypersexuality, by their definition, did not show any predictive value. The authors hypothesized that hypersexuality on its own does not lead to sexual offending but must be associated with antisociality or sexual deviance, as suggested by Mann et al. (2010). Again, the role of a CSBD or HD diagnosis was not specifically examined.

Another linked concept that has some overlap with CSBD and HD is sexual preoccupation. Brouillette-Alarie et al. (2016) found that rapists, but not child molesters, had higher sexual preoccupation. This was one of the relevant factors in the persistence/paraphilia construct that correlated with sexual recidivism. However, sexual deviance appeared to have most of the influence in this construct. The role of CSBD and HD was not specifically examined.

Although this evidence suggests that hypersexuality and related issues of sexual self-regulation problems, drive for impersonal sex, and compulsive masturbation are not relevant in recidivism, they do have a base in several multifactorial theories and developmental models of sexually coercive behavior (Malamuth 2003; Ward et al. 2006). Furthermore, a number of studies suggest that these issues do have relevance to reoffending. Hanson and Harris (2000) identified sexual preoccupation (generally defined as recurrent sexual thoughts or behaviors directed toward numerous casual or impersonal sexual encounters) as one of the most important dynamic risk factors for sexual offending, a finding that was replicated by Hanson et al. (2007). In one of the most recent and comprehensive meta-analyses of adult male sexual offenders, Hanson and Morton-Bourgon (2005) found that sexual preoccupation was significantly associated with sexual recidivism ($d=0.39$) and any violent recidivism ($d=0.28$).

Kingston and Bradford (2013) showed that individuals defined as "hypersexual" in their study were more likely to reoffend with either a sexual or violent offense than those who were not considered hypersexual. In terms of predictive accuracy, total sexual outlet was a moderate individual predictor of recidivism, and the effect was similar to results reported in a previous study (Knight and Thornton 2007) and a meta-analysis (Hanson and Morton-Bourgon 2005). These results support the notion that hypersexuality, and thus CSBD and HD, may be an important risk factor for sexually violent recidivism (Mann et al. 2010).

Ultimately, experts must know how to perform comprehensive risk assessments, including considering all validated variables relevant to the case. In criminal cases, structured professional judgment approaches may be helpful, such as the Risk for Sexual Violence Protocol (Hart et al. 2003), Stable-2007 (Hanson et al. 2007), and Sexual Violence Risk–20 (Boer et al. 1997), all of which consider relevant factors for sexual offending, including hypersexuality.

In psychiatric practice, it is also the norm to do a comprehensive biopsychosocial formulation in which the predisposing, precipitating, perpetuating, and protective factors in the biological, psychological, and social realms are analyzed to help understand patients' difficulties. This is similar to case conceptualization. It is important to thoroughly analyze all factors relevant to patients' sexual behavior. Individuals with hypersexuality may have a biologically higher sexual drive. Alternatively, they may use sexual behavior as a "self-soothing" outlet for stress. Many individuals whose sexual behavior causes legal issues have disordered lives (Fedoroff 2003); they frequently have problems with employment and with social, family, and marital relationships as well as comorbid difficulties with substance use, mood disorders, and anxiety disorders. It is important to evaluate all factors relevant to the behavior in order to assess the risk of further difficulties in the future.

Treatment of Hypersexuality

Often, legal decision makers are interested not only in the cause of the sexual behavior but also in its treatability. Therefore, experts must have a thorough and accurate understanding of the cause of offending and the treatable issues that might contribute. Marshall and Briken (2010) noted that diagnosis and assessment are important steps prior to initiating appropriate treatment of hypersexuality. In some cases, addressing non-hypersexual disorders may be the mainstay of treatment; for example, mood-stabilizing medication may be the primary treatment and very effective if the behavior was due to mania (Heare et al. 2016). Rivastigmine treatment of hypersexuality due to dementia has also been shown to be effective (Canevelli et al. 2013). In other cases, hypersexuality or CSBD may be a significant problem. Unfortunately, quality studies on specific interventions for hypersexuality and CSBD are very limited. Psychotherapeutic interventions have shown some effectiveness (Franqué et al. 2015). Cognitive-behavioral interventions are likely to be useful.

No medications are currently approved for the treatment of hypersexuality and CSBD. As such, all medications are used off-label, and prescribing would be based on theoretical benefits or limited clinical trials and clinical experience. Despite this, Kafka (2000) recommended pharmacological interventions for nonparaphilic hypersexuality, including use of serotonin reuptake inhibitors, dopamine agonists, and antiandrogen medications. Since then, gonadotropin-releasing hormone (GnRH) agonists have also been reported to be helpful for hypersexuality (Safarinejad 2009). Kaplan and Krueger (2010) reviewed the limited evidence for treatment of hypersexuality and highlighted similar medications as potentially helpful.

While almost no studies have specifically focused on the treatment of hypersexuality and CSBD, there are guidelines for treating patients with paraphilic disorders and sexual offending (Booth 2009; Thibaut et al. 2010). Presumably, some of this population would have hypersexuality or CSBD. There may also be overlap of the disorders, with similar response rates. Turner et al. (2014) suggested treatment for hypersexuality based on these guidelines.

Although literature on hypersexuality treatment is limited, it is reasonable to consider similar treatment modalities aimed at sexual offending. Again, a biopsychosocial approach can be effective. Many patients with hypersexuality note an obsessive quality to their sexual interests. Indeed, CSBD has been included as an impulse-control disorder in the ICD-11. Applying algorithms for treatment of sexual offending (Booth 2009) would likely be reasonable, assuming the risks of the intervention are balanced with the benefits. Thus, if the hypersexual behavior were increasingly dysfunctional, one could consider

- Serotonergic antidepressants as first line (e.g., sertraline 50–150 mg/day, paroxetine 20–40 mg/day, or similar)
- Augmenting agents (e.g., naltrexone 100–200 mg/day or psychostimulants such as methylphenidate up to 1 mg/kg/day)
- "Low-level" antitestosterone agents such as α-reductase inhibitors (e.g., finasteride 5 mg/day)
- Low-dose oral medroxyprogesterone acetate 50 mg/day or cyproterone acetate 50 mg/day
- High-dose oral medroxyprogesterone acetate 100–600 mg/day or cyproterone acetate 100–500 mg/day
- In extreme cases, intramuscular GnRH agonists such as leuprolide 7.5 mg/month, goserelin 3.6 mg/month, or triptorelin 3.75 mg/month)

Arguably, these approaches may have more success in hypersexuality and CSBD than with paraphilic interests because their mechanisms of action all primarily serve to decrease libido. Because they all would be considered off-label, with little empirical evidence, it would be vital to look at the risks and decide if the dysfunction justifies these interventions. In our clinical experience, these medications can be quite helpful. Some individuals notice a remarkable decrease in libido such that they can push down sexual urges. Serotonergic medications can also induce ejaculatory delay and anorgasmia. Although an unpleasant side effect for most patients, over time, individuals with hypersexuality become frustrated and bored with sexual activities that are no longer as satisfying, and many report seeking out other, more interesting activities of a nonsexual nature. Interestingly, 6 months to 1 year after beginning a selective serotonin reuptake inhibitor (SSRI), some patients seem to be able to taper their medication without a resurgence of hypersexuality. This suggests a possible behavioral component that extinguishes over time. Other patients note that as the SSRI decreases, their hypersexuality returns, and they would need to continue it longer term. Some patients may need to escalate to testosterone blockage, although the risk of more significant adverse effects increases.

In addition to biological factors, it is important to consider other psychosocial influences on offending. Much of the offender literature focuses on the risk-need-responsivity model (Bonta and Andrews 2007), but this approach does not easily lend itself to assessing and treating individuals with hypersexuality. The Good Lives Model (Marshall et al. 2005; Siegert et al. 2007; Ward and Gannon 2006) and related patient-centered approaches focus on helping sexual offenders live happier and more balanced lives, such that their need to use sex as an escape decreases. This includes helping patients maximize their satisfaction in employment, relationships, alone time and hobbies, social networks, emotional health, and other vital areas. Conceptualizing hypersexuality and CSBD as partly related to self-soothing and an escape from life problems, this approach would hold promise. These models often involve group work, wherein similar individuals can share their insights, strategies, and successes, thus helping each other further improve their overall function.

Although many potential treatments are available, further research is needed to clarify which interventions can be helpful for those with legal issues stemming from their hypersexuality. It is also important to be aware of the potential abuses of such interventions. A misplaced understanding of hypersexuality and sexual offending could result in courts mandating "chemical castration" or surgical castration. Indeed, history is full of reprehensible stories of so-called sexual deviants being forced to undergo castration—including those with homosexual interests, which we now consider nonpathological. As such, ethical practitioners ensure that any individuals presenting for treatment of their sexual issues are doing so with noncoerced informed consent.

At times, we have been asked to provide "court-ordered treatment" of sexual disorders. Court orders can range from requiring individuals to attend a psychotherapy group for sexual issues to requiring them to take a GnRH agonist, with treatment being a condition of freedom. Experts must inform the court that care providers cannot be ordered to provide treatment or to give medically unsafe treatments; indeed, a patient who does not want treatment is unlikely to benefit from a group therapy. Similarly, a patient's physical health might make certain medications dangerous. Instead, the court could order individuals to have an assessment and obtain treatment as recommended by the treatment provider. This allows for proper clinical evaluation.

Although such an approach may provide flexibility, courts may still seek to make treatment a condition of freedom. Providing treatment in such a situation must be done carefully. Many patients can competently assess the risks and benefits of treatment and reasonably want treatment to obtain the benefits (including freedom), but it is questionable whether their consent is being given without coercion under such circumstances. If it appears that coercion is the main motivation, the treating clinician should not participate.

EXPERT WITNESS ROLE

Forensic clinicians are often asked to serve as expert witnesses for the courts. The main goal is to educate the courts and decision makers about the motivation for an individual's behavior, the potential for treatment, and the risk of ongoing behavior. This includes cases of hypersexuality. Courts and tribunals often have special rules that allow experts to give opinion evidence, recognizing the risks of doing so (Booth et al. 2019). Other jurisdictions have similar criteria for the admissibility of novel-science evidence. Arguably, the construct of CSBD does not meet either *Frye* or *Daubert* criteria (described in the following paragraph). Novel science—areas that may have validity but have not been confirmed by evidence—is one of the special areas of law involving expert witness testimony. As discussed here and in other chapters, controversy remains in the literature about the diagnoses of HD and CSBD. As such, it could be argued that the diagnosis, treatment, and risk assessment of individuals with hypersexual behavior could still be considered novel science. The courts have examined this issue with concern that incorrect theories and "junk science" could be put forward as true.

The risk of novel science was first examined by U.S. courts in a case known as *Frye v. United States* (1923). The court ultimately said that new science put forward must be generally accepted in the field to be considered valid. U.S. courts evaluated this further in another case, known as *Daubert v. Merrell Dow Pharmaceuticals Inc.* (1993). This resulted in the *Daubert* criteria, which guide courts on whether to accept novel science. These criteria are as follows:

- Whether the theory or technique can be and has been tested
- Whether the theory or technique has been subjected to peer review and publication
- The known or potential rate of error or the existence of standards
- Whether the theory or technique used has been generally accepted

In Canada, the court looked at these issues in a case called *R. v. Mohan* (1994). For evidence to come into the court, it must be relevant and necessary for the fact finder, be given by a properly qualified expert, and be subject to an exclusionary rule. In another case, *R. v. J. (L.-J.)* (2000), the

Canadian courts confirmed that when looking at novel science, the criteria from *R. v. Mohan* plus the *Daubert* criteria should be applied (Glancy and Bradford 2007).

With this background, Marshall and Briken (2010) commented on the lack of general acceptance in the literature around the diagnosis of hypersexuality. They also highlighted the lack of high-quality studies to aid recommendations in this area. Thus, judges may rightfully decide to exclude testimony about a hypersexuality diagnosis.

Beyond novel science, other general principles for expert testimony are relevant to hypersexuality and CSBD. When called upon for such expertise, experts should consider several guiding questions:

- Are you qualified to perform such an assessment—do you have training and experience in mental disorders, neuropsychiatric disorders, pharmacology, and sexual issues, including hypersexuality and sexual offending?
- Do you have all information necessary for the evaluation to come to an opinion with a reasonable degree of medical certainty?
- Have you considered all potential driving and mitigating factors?
- Is there a "rational" explanation for the behavior, and have you discussed this?
- Have you been aware of and mentioned any potential biases and countertransference and any potential weaknesses in your information base?
- Have you avoided common expert witness mistakes?
- Have you highlighted areas of controversy in the field, including areas of novel science and lack of general acceptance?

SUMMARY AND CONCLUSIONS

We have outlined several important issues relevant for approaching the forensic aspects of hypersexuality. Practitioners must approach cases wherein hypersexuality may be an issue in an organized and evidence-based manner, with the goal of providing an accurate and legally defensible opinion. Forensic experts must be aware of the numerous potential mimics of hypersexuality, including neuropsychiatric disorders, psychiatric disorders, and medication-induced states. When presented with cases of inappropriate or concerning sexual behavior, some individuals may have hypersexuality at play; this may then enter administrative, civil, criminal, or family law and serve as a mitigating or aggravating factor or inform risk.

Ultimately, forensic experts must be careful in their role in educating the court and ensure that they are providing balanced testimony and opinions that are supported by the literature. They must also be fair, objective, and nonpartisan. In the case of hypersexuality, it is important to highlight the current controversies, lack of consensus in diagnosis, and mixed data around relevance to risk assessment.

References

American Psychiatric Association: Diagnostic and Statistical Manual of Mental Disorders, 5th Edition. Arlington, VA, American Psychiatric Association, 2013

Boer DP, Hart SD, Kropp PR, et al: Manual for the Sexual Violence Risk–20. Professional Guidelines for Assessing Risk of Sexual Violence. Vancouver, BC, Canada, Institute Against Family Violence, 1997

Bonta J, Andrews DA: Risk-Need-Responsivity Model for Offender Assessment and Rehabilitation. Ottawa, ON, Canada, Her Majesty the Queen in Right of Canada, 2007

Booth BD: How to select pharmacologic treatments to manage recidivism risk in sex offenders. Curr Psychiatry 8:60–72, 2009

Booth BD: Special populations: mentally disordered sexual offenders, in Managing High-Risk Sex Offenders in the Community: Risk Management, Treatment and Social Responsibilities. Edited by Harrison K. Devon, UK, Willan Publishing, 2010, pp 193–208

Booth BD: Legal issues involved in the management of paraphilic disorders, in Practical Guide to Paraphilia and Paraphilic Disorders. Edited by Balon R. Cham, Switzerland, Springer, 2016, pp 243–264

Booth BD, Gulati S: Mental illness and sexual offending. Psychiatr Clin North Am 37:183–194, 2014

Booth BD, Kingston DA: Sex offender risk assessment and management. Psychiatr Clin North Am 39:675–689, 2016

Booth BD, Schmedlen G: Sexually violent predator laws. J Am Acad Psychiatry Law 34:553–555, 2006

Booth BD, Watts J, Dufour M: Lessons from Canadian courts for all expert witnesses. J Am Acad Psychiatry Law 47(3):278–285, 2019

Bradford JM, de Amorim Levin G, Booth BD, et al: Forensic assessment of sex offenders, in The American Psychiatric Association Publishing Textbook of Forensic Psychiatry, 3rd Edition. Edited by Gold LH, Frierson RL. Washington, DC, American Psychiatric Association Publishing, 2018, pp 341–356

Brouillette-Alarie S, Babchishin KM, Hanson RK, et al: Latent constructs of the Static-99R and Static-2002R: a three-factor solution. Assessment 23:96–111, 2016

Canevelli M, Talarico G, Tosto G, et al: Rivastigmine in the treatment of hypersexuality in Alzheimer disease. Alzheimer Dis Assoc Disord 27:287–288, 2013

Cantor JM, Klein C, Lykins A, et al: A treatment-oriented typology of self-identified hypersexuality referrals. Arch Sex Behav 42:883–893, 2013

Daubert v. Merrell Dow Pharmaceuticals Inc., 509 U.S. 579 (1993)

Davies C: Sexual taboos and social boundaries. Am J Sociol 87:1032–1063, 1982

Devinsky J, Sacks O, Devinsky O: Kluver-Bucy syndrome, hypersexuality, and the law. Neurocase 16:140–145, 2010

Etzler S, Eher R, Rettenberger M: Dynamic risk assessment of sexual offenders: validity and dimensional structure of the Stable-2007. Assessment 27(4):822–839, 2018

Fabian JM: Diagnosing and litigating hebephilia in sexually violent predator civil commitment proceedings. J Am Acad Psychiatry Law 39:496–505, 2011

Fedoroff JP: Paraphilic worlds, in Handbook of Clinical Sexuality for Mental Health Professionals. Edited by Levine SB. New York, Brunner-Routledge, 2003, pp 333–356

Fedoroff JP: Forensic and diagnostic concerns arising from the proposed DSM-5 criteria for sexual paraphilic disorder. J Am Acad Psychiatry Law 39:238–241, 2011

First MB: DSM-5 and paraphilic disorders. J Am Acad Psychiatry Law 42:191–201, 2014

First MB, Halon RL: Use of DSM paraphilia diagnoses in sexually violent predator commitment cases. J Am Acad Psychiatry Law 36:443–454, 2008

Frances A, First MB: Hebephilia is not a mental disorder in DSM-IV-TR and should not become one in DSM-5. J Am Acad Psychiatry Law 39:78–85, 2011a

Frances A, First MB: Paraphilia NOS, nonconsent: not ready for the courtroom. J Am Acad Psychiatry Law 39:555–561, 2011b

Frances A, Wollert R: Sexual sadism: avoiding its misuse in sexually violent predator evaluations. J Am Acad Psychiatry Law 40:409–416, 2012

Franqué F, Klein V, Briken P: Which techniques are used in psychotherapeutic interventions for nonparaphilic hypersexual behavior? Sex Med Rev 3:3–10, 2015

Frye v. United States, 293 F. F. 1013 (1923)

Glancy GD, Bradford JM: The admissibility of expert evidence in Canada. J Am Acad Psychiatry Law 35:350–356, 2007

Greenland C: Sex law reform in an international perspective: England and Wales and Canada. Bull Am Acad Psychiatry Law 11:309–330, 1983

Halpern AL: The proposed diagnosis of hypersexual disorder for inclusion in DSM-5: unnecessary and harmful. Arch Sex Behav 40:487–490, 2011

Hanson R, Harris AJ: Where should we intervene? Dynamic predictors of sexual assault recidivism. Criminal Justice and Behavior 27:6–35, 2000

Hanson RK, Morton-Bourgon KE: The characteristics of persistent sexual offenders: a meta-analysis of recidivism studies. J Consult Clin Psychol 73:1154–1163, 2005

Hanson RK, Harris AJR, Scott T-L, et al: Assessing the Risk of Sexual Offender on Community Supervision: The Dynamic Supervision Project. Corrections Research User Report. Ottawa, ON, Canada, Public Safety Canada, 2007

Hart SD, Jackson K, Watt KA, et al: The Risk for Sexual Violence Protocol (RSVP): Structured Professional Guidelines for Assessing Risk for Sexual Violence. Vancouver, BC, Canada, The Institute Against Family Violence, 2003

Heare MR, Barsky M, Faziola LR: A case of mania presenting with hypersexual behavior and gender dysphoria that resolved with valproic acid. Ment Illn 8:6546, 2016

Hook JN, Hook JP, Davis DE, et al: Measuring sexual addiction and compulsivity: a critical review of instruments. J Sex Marital Ther 36:227–260, 2010

Kafka M: Psychopharmacologic treatments for nonparaphilic compulsive sexual behaviors. CNS Spectr 5:49–59, 2000

Kafka MP: Hypersexual disorder: a proposed diagnosis for DSM-V. Arch Sex Behav 39(2):377–400, 2010

Kafka MP: What happened to hypersexual disorder? Arch Sex Behav 43(7):1259–1261, 2014

Kafka MP, Prentky RA: Preliminary observations of DSM-III-R Axis I comorbidity in men with paraphilias and paraphilia-related disorders. J Clin Psychiatry 55:481–487, 1994

Kaplan MS, Krueger RB: Diagnosis, assessment, and treatment of hypersexuality. J Sex Res 47:181–198, 2010

Kingston DA, Bradford JM: Hypersexuality and recidivism among sexual offenders. Sexual Addiction and Compulsivity 20:91–105, 2013

Knight RA, Thornton D: Evaluating and Improving Risk Assessment Schemes for Sexual Recidivism: A Long-Term Follow-Up of Convicted Sexual Offenders. Award Number 2003-WG-BX-1002. Washington, DC, U.S. Department of Justice, 2007

Kraus SW, Krueger RB, Briken P, et al: Compulsive sexual behaviour disorder in the ICD-11. World Psychiatry 17(1):109–110, 2018

Krueger RB, Kaplan MS: Disorders of sexual impulse control in neuropsychiatric conditions. Semin Clin Neuropsychiatry 5:266–274, 2000

Kühn S, Gallinat J: Neurobiological basis of hypersexuality, in International Review of Neurobiology. Edited by Zahr NM, Peterson ET. Cambridge MA, Academic Press, 2016, pp 67–83

Ley D, Brovko JM, Reid RC: Forensic applications of "sex addiction" in US legal proceedings. Curr Sex Health Rep 7:108–116, 2015

Malamuth NM: Criminal and noncriminal sexual aggressors: integrating psychopathy in a hierarchical-mediational confluence model. Ann NY Acad Sci 989:33–58, discussion 144–153, 2003

Mann RE, Hanson RK, Thornton D: Assessing risk for sexual recidivism: some proposals on the nature of psychologically meaningful risk factors. Sex Abuse 22:191–217, 2010

Marshall LE, Briken P: Assessment, diagnosis, and management of hypersexual disorders. Curr Opin Psychiatry 23:570–573, 2010

Marshall WL, Ward T, Mann RE, et al: Working positively with sexual offenders: maximizing the effectiveness of treatment. J Interpers Viol 20:1096–1114, 2005

Montgomery-Graham S: Disorder in the court: the approach to sex addiction in Canadian legal proceedings. Canadian Journal of Human Sexuality 26:205–215, 2017

Novak B, McDermott BE, Scott CL, et al: Sex offenders and insanity: an examination of 42 individuals found not guilty by reason of insanity. J Am Acad Psychiatry Law 35:444–450, 2007

R. v. J.-L.J., 2 S.C.R. 600 (2000)

R. v. Mohan, 2 S.C.R. 9 (1994)

Reid RC, Kafka MP: Controversies about hypersexual disorder and the DSM-5. Curr Sex Health Rep 6:259–264, 2014

Reid RC, Garos S, Fong T: Psychometric development of the Hypersexual Behavior Consequences scale. J Behav Addict 1:115–122, 2012

Safarinejad MR: Treatment of nonparaphilic hypersexuality in men with a long-acting analog of gonadotropin-releasing hormone. J Sex Med 6:1151–1164, 2009

Siegert RJ, Ward T, Levack WM, et al: A good lives model of clinical and community rehabilitation. Disabil Rehabil 29:1604–1615, 2007

Steel C: The Asperger's defence in digital child pornography investigations. Psychiatry, Psychology and Law 23:473–482, 2016

Thibaut F, De La Barra F, Gordon H, et al: The World Federation of Societies of Biological Psychiatry (WFSBP) Guidelines for the biological treatment of paraphilias. World J Biol Psychiatry 11(4):604–655, 2010

Turner D, Schottle D, Bradford J, et al: Assessment methods and management of hypersexuality and paraphilic disorders. Curr Opin Psychiatry 27:413–422, 2014

Ward T, Gannon TA: Rehabilitation, etiology, and self-regulation: the comprehensive Good Lives model of treatment for sexual offenders. Aggression and Violent Behavior 11:77–94, 2006

Ward T, Polaschek DLL, Beech AR: Theories of Sexual Offending. Hoboken, NJ, Wiley, 2006

World Health Organization: International Classification of Diseases and Related Health Problems, 11th Revision. Geneva, World Health Organization, 2019

Zonana H: Sexual disorders: new and expanded proposals for the DSM-5—do we need them? J Am Acad Psychiatry Law Online 39:245–249, 2011

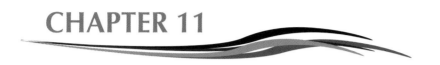

CHAPTER 11

Hypersexuality and Sexual Compulsivity

BEHAVIORAL/SEXUAL RISKS AND RISKS OF SEXUALLY TRANSMITTED DISEASES

Richard Balon, M.D.

This chapter addresses two important areas of research and the clinical care of persons with hypersexuality/compulsive sexual behavior disorder (CSBD): risky general and sexual behaviors and the possibility of increased prevalence of sexually transmitted diseases (STDs). Enough evidence indicates that hypersexuality is associated with various risky sexual and nonsexual behaviors and associated psychopathology. The association between hypersexuality and STDs is rather tenuous due to the lack of research in this area. The chapter also advocates for a focus on prevention and for awareness of the possibility of STDs among persons with hypersexuality/CSBD who seek clinical care.

RISK AND RISKY BEHAVIOR

A variety of behaviors and disorders may be associated with unwanted consequences. In other words, individuals with some disorders or behavioral features are *at risk* of developing mostly negative sequelae or consequences of their behavior. Hypersexuality and CSBD seem to be frequently associated with risky sexual behaviors. I refer to *risk* as a probability or likelihood that a certain event (usually a negative one) or disease will happen. Risk does not necessarily imply etiology but rather an association.

Risky sexual behavior is behavior that increases the chance a person who engages in sexual activity with another person will become infected with an STD if the partner has one, will get injured, will get pregnant, or will start using illicit drugs to enhance sexual enjoyment. More specifically, risky sexual behaviors include unprotected sex (which here means mainly not wearing condoms), multiple sexual partners, and legal or illicit substance use, such as alcohol, cocaine, marijuana, methamphetamine, opioids (especially intravenous), and others. The STDs include chlamydia, genital herpes, gonorrhea, hepatitis B, HIV/AIDS, syphilis, and trichomoniasis.

Unfortunately, most research of risky behavior and hypersexuality or sexual compulsivity has been done in studying risky behavior in homosexual men—that is, men who have sex with other men. Most of the research of risky behavior and STDs has also been done in this population. We need more research on associated behavioral risks and risks of STDs in heterosexual men and in both hetero- and homosexual women with CSBD.

CONCEPT OF SEXUAL SENSATION SEEKING

Increased risk associated with certain sexual behavior could be related to sexual sensation seeking. *Sensation seeking* is an old concept based on the construct of achieving an optimal level of stimulation or of arousal, since the "arousal construct could accommodate stimulus parameters such as novelty versus constancy, and complexity" (Zuckerman et al. 1978, p. 139). Conceptualized as a personality trait, sensation seeking has four factors:

- Thrill and adventure seeking: expressing a desire to engage in sports or other activities involving speed or danger

- Experience seeking: desire for new experiences through the mind and senses, travel, and nonconforming lifestyles
- Disinhibition: desire for social and sexual disinhibition expressed in social drinking, partying, and variety in sex partners
- Boredom susceptibility: aversion to repetition and routine and dullness and restlessness when things are unchanging

The initial concept of sensation seeking (Zuckerman et al. 1978) was later developed by Kalichman and colleagues (Kalichman and Rompa 1995; Kalichman et al. 1994, 1996), who considered Zuckerman's concept outdated. They proposed that a person takes various risks in order to enhance sexual behavior (Burri 2017). Kalichman and Rompa (1995) thought that sexual sensation-seeking behavior, as measured by their scale, corresponded to an attraction to various sexual practices, such as increased frequency of unprotected intercourse and greater number of sexual partners. Kalichman et al. (1996) also thought that, in addition to engagement in high-risk sexual practices, sensation seeking may mediate the association between substance abuse and risky sex. Thus, they proposed that assessing sexual sensation seeking may be useful for predicting sexual risk, such as for AIDS infection, and used in prevention of these behaviors and decreasing risks.

The etiology (genetic? psychological? social? biological [dopaminergic system]?) and relationship of sexual sensation seeking to sexual functioning, other clinical issues, sexual compulsivity, and hypersexuality have not been extensively or properly studied in recent years. However, in an interesting online study of 279 subjects in Switzerland, Burri (2017) found that in women, high levels of sexual sensation seeking were associated with higher levels of desire, arousal, lubrication, and orgasm and less sexual pain; no moderating effect of gender identity was detected. In men, sexual sensation seeking was significantly correlated with better ejaculatory function, and sexual compulsivity was correlated with worse erectile function.

It seems plausible that the personality trait of sexual sensation seeking plays a role in increasing the risk of various sexual behaviors (e.g., frequent sexual partners, lack of condom use, and other [substance use]) in individuals with CSBD or even in those who do not meet criteria for the disorder yet frequently engage in hypersexual behavior. It is not clear whether sexual sensation-seeking behavior increases the risk or mediates the association between risky behaviors and risky sexual behavior and hypersexuality. Nevertheless, sexual sensation seeking may play an important role in these highly intertwined risks and behaviors. It is also plausible that the increased frequency of sex with different partners (unless using protection, such as condoms) may lead to increased chance of acquiring some of the STDs.

Risky Behaviors and Hypersexuality

A number of studies have examined risky behaviors—nonsexual, sexual, and related to STDs (mostly infection with HIV)—in relationship to hypersexuality (but not to CSBD, because that diagnosis has become official only recently). These studies examined either hypersexuality or sexual compulsivity (because they are used interchangeably, I use them this way), almost exclusively in men. Some studies reported risky sexual behaviors, some reported risky nonsexual behaviors that could be related to sexual behavior, and some reported both.

Predominantly Sexual Risky Behavior

In 1999, Benotsch and colleagues, in their sample of 112 HIV-seropositive men who had sex with men, observed that men scoring high on sexual compulsivity reported engaging in more frequent unprotected sexual acts with more partners, reported greater use of cocaine in conjunction with sexual activity, rated high-risk sexual acts as more pleasurable, and reported lower self-esteem. Interestingly, mediational analyses indicated that both personal and partner use of cocaine partially mediated the relationship between sexual compulsivity and high-risk sexual behavior. Similarly, Semple et al. (2006) reported various risky sexual behaviors (and some nonsexual risks) in a sample of 217 HIV-positive methamphetamine-using homosexual and bisexual men in San Diego, California, including using methamphetamines before and during sex, visiting sex clubs and street corners to find sex partners, and having a greater number of HIV-negative or unknown serostatus partners, as well as lower self-efficacy for condom use, higher scores on a measure of disinhibition, and lower self-esteem.

A complex risky behavior—serodiscordant unprotected anal intercourse—was independently associated with use of stimulants, poppers, alcohol, and erectile dysfunction medications and sexual compulsivity in a probability sample of 711 men who had sex with men (Woolf-King et al. 2013). The association of this complex risky behavior and sexual compulsivity was moderated by poppers and erectile dysfunction medication. In a small Brazilian study (Scanavino et al. 2013) of 86 men (26% homosexual, 17% bisexual, 57% heterosexual) who met criteria for excessive sexual drive and sexual addiction, homosexual and bisexual men were more likely to report casual sex and sex with multiple casual partners as problematic behaviors. In another study (Parsons et al. 2016), 370 highly sexually active homosexual and bisexual men were divided into three groups: no sexual compulsivity and no hypersexual disorder (48.9%), sexual compulsivity only (30%), and both sexual compulsivity and hypersexual disorder (21.1%). Men in the combined sexual compulsivity and hypersexual disorder group reported higher numbers of condomless anal sex and condomless anal sex with serodiscordant partners than did men in the sexual compulsivity–only group.

In a cross-sectional study of self-identified 436 homosexual and bisexual men in Southwest China, Xu et al. (2016) found that sexual sensation seeking, sexual compulsivity, and sexual attitude (measured by the Sexual Attitude Scale, drawn from the Sociosexual Orientation Inventory) were associated with having male casual sexual partners and unprotected anal intercourse with multiple casual sexual partners.

Predominantly Nonsexual Risky Behavior and Psychopathology

Langström and Hanson (2006) studied 2,450 men and women from a 1996 national survey of sexuality and health in Sweden to examine the risk factors of hypersexuality in a representative, nonclinical population. Hypersexual men (N=151; 12.1% of all male subjects) reported engaging in a number of risky behaviors such as smoking tobacco, heavy drinking, using illegal drugs, and gambling. They were relatively less satisfied with their physical and psychological health and with life in general. For hypersexual women (N=80; 7% of all female subjects) the correlates were substantially the same; however, in contrast to men, hypersexuality in women was related to increased psychiatric morbidity. Psychiatric comorbidity has been a confounding variable in other studies, but in a different direction; for instance, in the Scanavino et al. (2013) study of 86 homosexual, bisexual, and heterosexual men, Sexual Compulsivity Scale (Kalichman and Rompa 2001) scores were associated with psychiatric comorbidities, mood disorder, and suicide risk.

Further exploring personality factors and behavioral mechanisms relevant to hypersexuality in men who have sex with men, Miner et al. (2016) compared 93 men assigned to hypersexuality and 143 nonhypersexual men using a number of scales and other instruments (group assignment was based on a Structured Clinical Interview for DSM–type interview). The authors found that hypersexuality was related to two personality factors characterized by emotional reactivity, risk taking, and impulsivity. There was a positive relationship between hypersexuality and negative emotionality and a negative relationship with constraint.

SEXUALLY TRANSMITTED DISEASES AND HYPERSEXUALITY

Intuitively, risky sexual behavior, such as having multiple partners or having unprotected sex with multiple partners, should be associated with increased chance of becoming infected with STDs. However, interestingly, the evidence for this association in the literature is scarce. A PubMed search (as of October 2020) did not reveal any publication on the possible association of chlamydia, gonorrhea, hepatitis B, or trichomoniasis with hypersexuality.

In the National Survey of Sexual Attitudes and Lifestyles, Johnson et al. (2001) interviewed a probability sample of 4,762 men and 6,399 women ages 16–44 in Great Britain. They noted that the prevalence of many reported sexual behaviors had risen compared with data from a similar survey done in 1990 and that the increased reporting of risky sexual behaviors was consistent with changing cohabitation patterns and the rising incidence of STDs (infections unspecified). The range of behaviors associated with increased risk of HIV and STDs included number of sexual partners, homosexual partnership, concurrent partnership, heterosexual anal sex, and payment for sex. However, this study did not explore hypersexuality as one of the factors, and thus any conclusion about association of hypersexuality and STDs mediated by risky sexual behavior is only speculative.

Turban et al. (2017) studied 283 postdeployment U.S. combat veterans regarding their digital social media use for seeking sexual partners. The use of digital social media to find sexual partner status (79 veterans, 70 men and 7 women) was positively associated with number of lifetime and annual sexual partners, recent casual sex (past 30 days), STDs, and hypersexuality. The relationship between hypersexuality and STDs was not clarified, and its existence via mediation with using digital social media for seeking sexual partners is again speculative.

Two studies addressed the possible relationship between hypersexuality and HIV infection/transmission. Moskowitz et al. (2011) conducted a large survey ($N=1,554$) at one leather and one nonleather event, collecting data from 655 subjects who identified as submissives, dominants, switches, and nonorienting leathermen. Leathermen are a self-defined subculture that has a heightened valuation of hypersexuality and adherence to sexual control dynamics such as submission and dominance. Leathermen were 61% more likely to be HIV positive than nonleathermen. A possible factor contributing to heightened HIV rates was decreased condom use among HIV-positive leathermen compared with

HIV-positive nonleathermen. Similarly, Grov et al. (2014b) compared three cohorts of sexually active men who have sex with men: 50 men recruited through Craigslist, 48 men recruited in gay bars and clubs, and 50 men recruited via private sex-party promoters. Men recruited from sex parties reported more symptoms of sexual compulsivity (highest score on Sexual Compulsivity Scale), were more likely to be HIV positive (46%, highest of all three groups), more likely to report a history of STDs, and more likely to self-identify as a "barebacker" (i.e., not using condoms) than were men in the other two groups. As in other studies on STDs, the direct relation between hypersexuality and HIV status was not studied; conclusions were based on the fact that hypersexual men were more frequently infected with HIV.

An interesting case from India (Dutta and Naphade 2017) described a young hypersexual male who was diagnosed with syphilis (confirmed by rapid plasma reagin test). Considering the serious impact of STDs, some with fatal outcomes (e.g., HIV/AIDS, syphilis) and some with serious nonfatal consequences but impacts on physical health and interpersonal relationships, it is surprising how little research has been done on the relationship between hypersexuality and STDs. Most literature addresses the relationship between homosexual sex and STDs, namely HIV/AIDS, with the unspoken implication that hypersexuality plays a role in this relationship. That is simply an unacceptable conclusion from a scientific point of view. Although some homosexual persons, mainly men, display various risky sexual behaviors, this does not mean that all homosexual people are hypersexual. This issue must be addressed in studies that examine STD rates in subjects with diagnosed CSBD/hypersexuality and compare them with nonhypersexual homo- and heterosexual persons.

In the meantime, clinicians need to be vigilant for the possible presence of STDs in patients with CSBD, actively asking them about STDs and their symptoms and possibly using appropriate diagnostic testing. Medications for treating STDs (e.g., antivirals) could have significant interactions with other medications. Psychoeducation about STDs, medications, and risky behavior should be a part of treatment.

STD-preventive measures should always be part of the overall care for CSBD. Several studies have suggested the usefulness of targeting men who have sex with HIV- and STD-positive men with preventive measures such as

- Free lubricants and condoms as well as free rapid HIV testing at sex parties (Grov et al. 2014a);

- A focus on increasing outcome expectancies for condom use, HIV disclosure, and negotiation of safer sex practices (Brown et al. 2016);
- Cognitive-behavioral therapy tailored for HIV-positive subjects based on the Unified Protocol for the Transdiagnostic Treatment of Emotional Disorders (Parsons et al. 2017); and
- A combination of HIV self-testing with patient-delivered partner therapy and partner notification via an application (John et al. 2020).

Mr. J

Mr. J, a 26-year-old single male, was referred to a psychiatrist by his primary care physician, who was concerned about Mr. J's low self-esteem, poor impulse control, anger, and admission of having multiple sexual partners and being treated for a number of STDs, including gonorrhea (twice), chlamydia, and genital herpes.

During the initial appointment, Mr. J was hesitant to discuss his sexuality and sexual behaviors at first but admitted to having multiple sexual partners ("nothing wrong with it at my age"), both female and male. He considered himself a "curious bisexual guy" who "enjoys sex immensely" and has to have it every day, preferably more than once a day. It was difficult for him to find a partner who would satisfy his desire for multiple sexual encounters daily; experimentations with sexual enhancers, such as a low dose of cocaine ("just one line"); and bisexuality ("you would not believe the jealousness of some of my lovers"). Thus, he had been frequenting various gay parties and had sought sex with female sex workers.

Mr. J was the only child of two successful professionals. His father is a lawyer, and his mother worked as a manager for a large shipping company. He described his childhood as "fairly normal, uneventful," except for his father's bouts of drinking and occasional fights between his parents: "My mother was always suspicious that my father had affairs with his clients, but he always denied it and nothing has ever been confirmed." Mr. J graduated from a prestigious local college and obtained a master of business administration degree. He started to work in a managerial position in an automotive company. He liked his work, and his pay allowed him a comfortable lifestyle. However, he did not think that his parents fully appreciated his education and good job, saying "they always suggest that I wasted my talent by not becoming a doctor or a lawyer. It does not feel good to hear this all the time." He also did not feel "part of the crowds" at work: "Most of the guys are married or are getting married; they have different interests, keep asking me about my dates. They are typical corporate guys." He had been feeling lonely in spite of his frequent dates and sexual encounters.

Mr. J said that he had always been interested in sex, as long as he could remember: "I have always found sex very exciting." When he was 12 years old, he learned that his father was occasionally watching pornographic videos. "It was fascinating, new, exciting...and I watched it, too, when nobody else was at home." He started to masturbate while watching pornography. Around the age of 14, he had his first sexual intercourse with "a bit older girl from the neighborhood." "We liked each other, and sex was good, but then her brother found out and told her that she should not have sex with a kid." Mr. J started to have sex with other girls from his high school and his neighborhood. "I kept it secret, though I had many girls." At college, he became sexually attracted to a male classmate who made some advances toward him. "It surprised me first, but then I said to myself, why not?, and I found sex with him very exciting." He considered himself bisexual but said that sex with women "is less complicated; they are less domineering." He had been using condoms during sex with men only because he was afraid of HIV infection, "but women do not have AIDS, I don't use condoms when having sex with them. Sex with a condom on is less pleasurable, less exciting." He masturbated on days when there were no sexual partners available. When asked about substance use, he stated that he rarely drank alcohol, did not smoke, and used small amounts of cocaine only in the context of sex, "to make it better."

After the initial consultation, Mr. J was given psychoeducation about STDs, especially about the necessity of using a condom with casual partners of both sexes. He accepted the offer of HIV testing and was found to be negative. He started a combination of supportive and cognitive-behavioral therapy that focused on his low self-esteem, mild depression, loneliness, risky behaviors, and inability to establish a long-lasting relationship. Because he continued to be mildly depressed and focused on satisfying his high sexual desire, he was prescribed 10 mg of fluoxetine, and it was explained to him that fluoxetine may lower his libido. The dosage was later increased to 20 mg/day. His mood improved and his sexual desire decreased. The number of his sexual encounters also decreased, although he continued to masturbate about once a day. He started to use condoms during all sexual encounters. A year later, Mr. J continued in therapy, working on his issues of relationships and loneliness. He felt happier, saying "Maybe I am on the right track." He had not acquired any STDs within the past year.

CONCLUSION

Hypersexuality seems to be associated with various risky sexual behaviors such as unprotected sex, more partners, use of cocaine in conjunction with sex (mediator) and use of methamphetamines, visits to sex clubs and street corners to find sex partners, low efficacy for condom use ("barebacking"), higher scores of disinhibition, and a high number of HIV-negative or unknown-serostatus partners. It also seems to be associated with low self-esteem, less satisfaction with psychological and physical health and life in general; risk taking in general; impulsivity, disinhibition, and emotional reactivity; and psychiatric comorbidity.

The relationship between hypersexuality and STDs has not been firmly established because it has not been well studied. The higher risk and prevalence of STDs in persons with hypersexuality is mostly presumed, based on their increased risky sexual behavior, such as sex with multiple partners and lack of using condoms. Nevertheless, the possibility of STDs in persons with hypersexuality/CSBD must be addressed in clinical encounters through psychoeducation, clinical examination, testing, and appropriate treatment and by the implementation and promotion of preventive measures.

Most research studies focusing on these areas have been done in homosexual subjects, mostly homosexual men, and thus we lack data on heterosexual men and heterosexual and homosexual women. We definitely need more research focused on risky behaviors and the prevalence of STDs in persons with hypersexuality/CSBD. Findings of such research may help us better advocate for establishing more prevention and treatment programs. Prevention programs seem to be especially important for STDs. It would also be interesting to see how much of today's research findings on hypersexuality will reflect on or "transfer" to research on tomorrow's CSBD.

REFERENCES

Benotsch EG, Kalichman SC, Kelly JA: Sexual compulsivity and substance use in HIV- seropositive men who have sex with men: prevalence and predictors of high-risk behaviors. Addict Behav 24:857–868, 1999

Brown MJ, Seriovich JM, Kimberly JA: Outcome expectancy and sexual compulsivity among men who have sex with men living with HIV. AIDS Behav 20:1667–1674, 2016

Burri A: Sexual sensation seeking, sexual compulsivity, and gender identity and its relationship with sexual functioning in a population sample of men and women. J Sex Med 14:69–77, 2017

Dutta E, Naphade NM: Hypersexuality—a case of concern: a case report highlighting the need for psychodermatology liaison. Indian J Sex Transm Dis AIDS 38:180–182, 2017

Grov C, Rendina HJ, Breslow AS, et al: Characteristics of men who have sex with men (MSM) who attend sex parties: results from a national online sample in the USA. Sex Trans Infect 90(1):26–32, 2014a

Grov C, Rendina HJ, Parsons JT: Comparing three cohorts of MSM sampled via sex parties, bars/clubs, and Craiglist.org: implications for researchers and providers. AIDS Educ Prev 26:362–382, 2014b

John SA, Starks TJ, Rendina HJ, Parsons JT: High willingness to use novel HIV and bacterial sexually transmitted infection partner notification, testing, and treatment strategies among gay and bisexual men. Sex Trans Infect 93:173–176, 2020

Johnson AM, Mercer KH, Erens B, et al: Sexual behaviour in Britain: partnership, practices, and HIV risk behaviours, Lancet 358:1835–1842, 2001

Kalichman SC, Rompa D: Sexual sensation seeking and sexual compulsivity scales: reliability, validity, and predicting HIV risk behavior. J Pers Assess 65(3):585–601, 1995

Kalichman SC, Rompa D: The Sexual Compulsivity Scale: further development and use with HIV-positive persons. J Pers Assess 76:379–395, 2001

Kalichman SC, Johnson JR, Adair V, et al: Sexual sensation seeking: scale development and predicting AIDS-risk behavior among homosexually active men. J Pers Assess 62:385–397, 1994

Kalichman SC, Heckman T, Kelly JA: Sensation seeking as an explanation for the association between substance use and HIV-related risky sexual behavior. Arch Sex Behav 25:141–154, 1996

Langström N, Hanson RK: High rates of sexual behavior in the general population: correlates and predictors. Arch Sex Behav 35:37–52, 2006

Miner MH, Romine RS, Raymond N, et al: Understanding the personality and behavioral mechanisms defining hypersexuality in men who have sex with men. J Sex Med 13:1323–1331, 2016

Moskowitz DA, Seal DW, Rintamaki L, Rieger G: HIV in the leather community: rates and risk-related behaviors. AIDS Behav 15:557–564, 2011

Parsons JT, Rendina HJ, Ventuneac A, Moody RL: Hypersexual, sexually compulsive, or just highly sexually active? Investigating three distinct groups of gay and bisexual men and their profiles of HIV-related sexual risk. AIDS Behav 20:262–272, 2016

Parsons JT, Rendina HJ, Moody RL, et al: Feasibility of an emotion regulation intervention to improve mental health and reduce HIV transmission risk behaviors for HIV-positive gay and bisexual men with sexual compulsivity. AIDS Behav 21:1540–1549, 2017

Scanavino MdT, Ventuneac A, Abdo CHN, et al: Compulsive sexual behavior and psychopathology among treatment-seeking men in Sao Paulo, Brazil. Psychiatry Res 209(3):518–524, 2013

Semple SJ, Zians J, Grant I, Patterson TL: Sexual compulsivity in a sample of HIV-positive methamphetamine-using gay and bisexual men. AIDS Behav 10(5):587–598, 2006

Turban J, Potenza MN, Hoff RA, et al: Psychiatric disorders, suicidal ideation, and sexually transmitted infections among post-deployment veterans who utilize digital social media for sexual partner seeking. Addict Behav 66:96–100, 2017

Woolf-King SE, Rice MT, Truong H-HM, et al: Substance use and HIV risk behavior among men who have sex with men: the role of sexual compulsivity. J Urban Health 90:948–952, 2013

Xu W, Zheng L, Liu Y, Zheng Y: Sexual sensation seeking, sexual compulsivity, and high-risk sexual behaviours among gay/bisexual men in Southwest China. AIDS Care 28:1138–1144, 2016

Zuckerman M, Eysenck S, Eysenck HJ: Sensation seeking in England and America: cross- cultural, age, and sex comparisons. J Consult Clin Psychol 46:139–149, 1978

CHAPTER 12

Religious and Cultural Influences of CSBD

António Pacheco Palha, M.D., Ph.D.
Mário Ferreira Lourenço, M.D., Ph.D.

Sexuality is natural to human life and an integral part of it, mainly involving pleasure, reproduction, and couple relationships. The definition of a sexual act varies considerably across cultures and even among people in the same culture; however, in all cultures and in all historical periods, some individuals develop compulsive sexual behavior (CSB). Compulsive sexual behavior disorder (CSBD) is a repetitive and intense preoccupation with sex; individuals with CSBD cannot manage their sexual behavior and experience significant distress as a result.

Culture plays a decisive role in coloring the pathology of various sexual disorders (Bhugra et al. 2010). The traditional values, beliefs, and practices of some indigenous peoples hold ancient wisdom regarding healing and healthy sexuality (Delugach 1999). The traditional sexual laws are a given because the person has the use of reason and is able to know what is prohibited and what allowed in his or her culture (Douglas 2003). Culture enriches and helps shape the expression of sexuality. When we approach the knowledge of the different forms of life and production of communities in their natural context, the harmonious relationship between cultures, their organization, their worldview, and the forms of territorial management appears with increasing clarity, always referring to an ethic, a concept of respect toward all beings who inhabit it and their spiritual owners (Battiste and Youngblood 2000). In indigenous cultures, behaviors—namely, in the area of sexuality—manifest their worldview; health is affected by the balance between the material and the spiritual, between nature and the body (Wilson 2003). The expression of some paraphilic disorders, such as cross-dressing in transvestic disorder, is influenced by the specific culture.

Current views on sexual health also have their roots in sexual abuse, sexual behaviors considered strange and nonconsensual, marital conflict, and sexual dysfunction. Indigenous models of healing and healthy sexuality can not only complement this body of knowledge but also connect sexuality with spirituality (Delugach 1999; Kirmayer et al. 2003). The understanding of appropriate sexual behavior tied to moderation and control has a long history. Western culture has always found it difficult to accept sexual behaviors that are not intended for procreation (Giddens 2013).

WHEN HISTORY AND CULTURE INFLUENCE EACH OTHER

Medicine in general, and psychiatry in particular, have always paid attention to hypersexual behavior. Richard von Krafft-Ebing, a nineteenth-century Western European pioneer sexologist, and Magnus Hirschfeld, working in the twentieth century, identified and characterized nymphomania and satyriasis as examples of excessive sexual behaviors in women and men, respectively (Bullough 1989; Hirschfeld 1948; von Krafft-Ebing 1998). Today, the clinical use of these terms is obsolete. *Satyriasis* was used to describe excessive or abnormal sexual craving in males; the corresponding term for females was *nymphomania*. In popular culture and European literature, satyriasis gained visibility thanks to some iconic characters, such as the Don Juan myth. Don Juan is an archetype of Spanish literature, a conqueror and seducer of women who collects them like trophies and then deceives and abandons them in search of the next woman. The characteristics of this seductive and libertine character created what in Western culture is known as Don Juanism, which is posited as a relationship between the sexes that gives men inconsiderate superiority over women. Since the first appearance of the myth, this figure has been instilled in the thinking and feeling of Western culture and identifies an insatiable male with an exacerbated and uncontrolled sexuality. In Don Juanism, men hunger for loving conquest, seeking only transitory enjoyment and the pride of triumph, whereas women lack defensive capacity (Alonso-Fernández 2002). This image of the seducer, of one who accumulates conquests and believes there is time for everything, is one vector of the myth (Pratt 1960).

Women with insatiable sexual appetites have been described since ancient Greece in the form of the famous nymphs, the gods propitiating reproduction. The word *nymphomania* comes from the Greek *nymphe* (young girl) and *mania* (obsession). The Roman empress Valeria Messalina and the Russian empress Catherine the Great were historical figures who, through their agitated love lives, made women's free sexual practice an element of affirmation and liberation (Berger 2002; Massie 2012; Ramazanoglu 1993). Women with nymphomania were often described as being devoid of self-will, slaves to their own desires. In 1771, French physician De Bienville published his treatise *La Nymphomanie, ou Traité de la Fureur Utérine*, giving birth to the idea of nymphomania as a moral perversion at a time when any small sexual transgression was enough to label a woman as "lost" and a public health menace (Boucé 1980).

Although mainly discredited now, demonology was also a factor in the conceptualization of hypersexuality for some medical theorists, even into the eighteenth century. It was believed that when one's sexual urge can no longer be controlled and assumes exaggerated and incalculable dimensions, it enters the dark depths of the soul, where the mind can exercise no influence and demons hold sway (Diethelm 1971).

Thus, in dominant culture and even in medical thinking, debauched people were viewed as having a disordered mind and prone to risky sexual behaviors that could ultimately lead to sexually transmitted diseases and mental and physical dissipation. von Krafft-Ebing stated that in the most extreme cases even death could result; in fact, in 1871, the psychiatrist Maresch documented three such cases in which the victims were said to have died of exhaustion because of their obscene delusions (Oosterhuis 2000). The author was probably describing some situations of erotomania and not so much of CSB.

Current research on hypersexual disorder focuses largely on men. In the psychiatric nosology, for a long time, nymphomania and satyriasis were confused with erotomania (Bellomo 2005). For Esquirol (1782–1840), however, erotomania differed essentially from nymphomania and satyriasis because in erotomania, love "was in the head" (*"l'amour est dans la tête"*), considering it an intellectual monomania—that is, a form of mental alignment that partially affects the mind, leaving the intellectual faculties intact, whose cause is a pathological passion that acts on the intelligence, fixing its attention. He called it the "madness of chaste love" (*folie de l'amour chaste*) (Berrios and Kennedy 2002; Esquirol et al. 1991; Sophia et al. 2007).

Cultures define and describe what is normal and what is deviant. In non-Western cultures, sex is no less stigmatized; gender discrimination prevails and mass media places sexual images and concepts into popular culture, raising unsound stereotypes of sexuality. Although the literature on sexual compulsivity is sparse, Morgan (2010) pointed out that Pakistan is one of the countries where the internet is most used to search for pornographic content. On the Indian subcontinent, for example, the weight of traditions and history mix with a modernity forced by economic development. Here one also finds the culture-bound *dhat syndrome* (Bhatia and Malik 1991), which is highly prevalent not only in India but also in its neighboring countries: Pakistan, Nepal, Myanmar, and Sri Lanka, among others. The word *dhat* derives from the Sanskrit word *dhatu* (which has multiple meanings including "metal," "elixir," and "constituent part of the body") (Kar and Sarkar 2015). Dhat syndrome is a clinical entity that includes a multitude of symptoms, both organic and psychological, attributed by patients to the passing of whitish fluid, believed to be semen, in their urine (i.e., psychological distress and anxiety related to semen loss) (Sumathipala et al. 2004). It may also include some symptoms associated with sexual compulsivity, such as frequent and uncontrolled masturbation. The phenomenon of globalization and routes of emigration explain the appearance of cases similar to dhat syndrome in other geographical regions, including Central Asia and Europe.

Strictly speaking, dhat syndrome is not a psychosexual dysfunction but a sexual-related disorder and is often considered a culture-specific sexual neurosis. In cultures in which fear of masturbation prevails, the urogenital system is the focus of concern. In traditional Ayurvedic medicine, all bodily secretions are highly purified (*dhatu*), namely, the urine, semen, and vaginal secretions; the loss of these body fluids results in a loss of vitality. "Excessive," "unnatural," or "immoral" semen loss can negatively impact health in general and sexual health in particular (Singh 1985). Sexual problems associated with excessive masturbation (especially sexual dysfunctions and intense negative feelings) are commonly reported on the Indian subcontinent; Nakra et al. (1977) found that nearly 43% of subjects had guilt associated with masturbation.

People with dhat syndrome amplify somatic symptoms and health-related anxiety by altering their perception of physiological signals, for example, the color of their urine or the loss of semen (Ranjith and Mohan

2004). They often complain of fatigue, without febrile movement and tenacious asthenia. Dhat syndrome presents with deep-set, shadowed eyes, a dull look, withered skin, an emaciated face, pronounced weight loss, and general suggestive aspect of premature aging (Ware and Weiss 1994). Patients' mood is gloomy and pessimistic, hypochondriacal complaints about their body prevail, and they experience a state of intellectual exhaustion, with difficulty concentrating, thinking, and speaking fluently (Behere and Natraj 1984). Because the syndrome relates to anxiety surrounding semen loss, it is (necessarily) found among men, but interestingly, it has also been considered in women who experience similar symptoms related to white vaginal discharge (Edwards 1983; Trollope-Kumar 2001).

We now present two clinical cases in which sexual compulsivity is modeled, conditioned, and "enriched" by the patients' cultural context, beliefs, and education. These are fictitious clinical cases in which any data that could identify the patients have been replaced or disguised.

CASE EXAMPLES

Mr. R

History of Present Illness

Mr. R was a 38-year-old married heterosexual male and father of two children who worked in the textile industry. He was referred by his general practitioner (GP) to the psychiatry outpatient department. He presented with chief complaints of pain in the genital region and an increased sexual desire over the past 16 years, accompanied by repeated masturbation. He desperately desired to stop. The intensity of the complaints had increased over the past 3 years; he had missed work for long periods and his marriage was in danger.

Mr. R reported having excessive and "out-of-control" masturbatory sexual behavior. In desperation, he gained courage and decided to ask his GP for help because he was not able to talk about it with anyone else. His other relevant symptoms included abusive alcohol consumption, insomnia, restlessness, anorexia, thoughts related to the fear of losing sexual function, and difficulties in social relationships. He reported his mood as sad and intensely anxious. He had ideas of hopelessness, helplessness, and worthlessness but no suicidal ideation. He did not show any mania-like or psychotic symptoms with sexual content and did not meet criteria for obsessive-compulsive symptomatology. He had no history of childhood sexual abuse and no environmental triggers for his sexual preoccupations.

Psychiatric History

Mr. R's psychiatric history included two periods of depressive episodes that occurred 6 years ago. He had been prescribed an antidepressant medication, sertraline 100 mg, by his GP, which he took for 11 months.

In the first interview, Mr. R felt quite embarrassed to approach matters related to his sex life. After some insistence, he finally admitted that in adolescence he had a high sexual appetite and masturbated with no feelings of guilt. Even after marrying, he usually masturbated 3–10 times a week and often masturbated before intercourse to sustain and control the strong sexual desire that overwhelmed his mind and body. For a period he and his wife had watched pornographic films before intercourse, and as a result of these stimuli, their sexual life improved slightly, with coital frequency increasing. However, this effect was relatively short-lived because, according to Mr. R, his wife "became bored with it."

After the birth of their two sons, everything changed. His wife gradually stopped taking the initiative in intercourse. She was always in a bad mood; she began to question him and was not satisfied with his detached behavior. Their emotional withdrawal and lack of communication had become two relevant characteristics in the life of this couple. Mr. R started masturbating nightly. Gradually, he started doing it even in the workplace. He had to masturbate four or five times a day and felt anxious if he did not do so. He claimed that if he stopped masturbating, he would not get sleep and would feel irritable and uneasy. He tried to divert his mind by listening to music or watching television but without any improvement. He said that due to this habit, his work performance had deteriorated; he was unable to concentrate and was always looking for a place to masturbate. His mind would be preoccupied with these obsessive thoughts throughout the day.

Past Sexual History

Issues related to sexuality were never addressed at home. Everything he knew about sexuality had been learned on the internet and through friends at school. Mr. R described his parents as being particularly religious, so naturally, religious practices influenced his own life choices, his behaviors, and the way he perceived the world around him. Curiously or not, Mr. R had never been able to confess his sexual problems to the priests of the churches he attended.

Since puberty, Mr. R liked to think about sex. This inclination increased in frequency, and from the age of 20 his friends began to say he was a "sexual pervert." When he saw a beautiful woman on the street, he would get excited and find a way to masturbate soon after. For him it was reasonable to "daydream," to fantasize about sexual relations, ending by quenching his libido through masturbation one to five times a day. Occasionally Mr. R used the internet to increase his degree of excitement, but he believed that "one good thought was worth a thousand images." Considering his low salary, he only rarely used prostitutes. He enjoyed these sexual activities, did not consider them abnormal, and could not abstain, although he admitted that they were excessive.

Discussion

The role of culture in the construction of desire is more real than often thought. Culturally and historically, religion has had a prominent effect on sexuality. Religiousness and sexual behavior are intricately related domains of human functioning. Higher degrees of religiosity are associated with negative attitudes toward nonprocreative sexual activities, guilt about masturbation, less likelihood of engaging in sexual intercourse, and fewer sex partners if sexually experienced (Nicholas 2004).

The moral emotion of shame increases when individuals have sexual practices that are considered nonconsensual, and those who are more spiritual or connected to God are less likely to have sex after consuming alcohol (Murray et al. 2007). Studies consistently demonstrate that hypersexuality is negatively related to measures of spiritual adjustment, and the manner in which this divergence is born has a clearly cultural mark (Karaga et al. 2016).

Religious beliefs can strongly influence appraisals of sexual behavior, especially to the degree that individuals view themselves as failing to act in line with their sexual values. Meanwhile, as the case of Mr. R demonstrates, they often paradoxically reinforce one another, as religious imagery, iconography, restraints, penances, the sublimation of personal needs, and spiritual devotion in some cases end up being invested with an erotic connotation. The impact of religiosity on sexuality depends essentially on the role and predisposition of the individual and suggests that the effects of religious group and sexual attitudes and fantasies may be mediated through individual differences. Mr. R's belief system, coupled with his personality (an obsessive trait) and marital difficulties, eventually influenced and shaped the way his sexuality manifested.

Mr. S

History of Present Illness

Mr. S, a 34-year-old male, was married with one son. He lived in an urban area and was from an upper-middle-class family. The only son of three children, he had been brought up in a conservative and rigid family in Angola. He had obtained his master's degree in computer engineering at the University of Minho in Guimarães, Portugal. He had sought psychiatric care 2 years ago, with the chief complaint of uncontrollable excessive watching of pornography. Other relevant symptoms included progressive and disturbing social isolation, pessimism, depressed mood, mistrustful ideas, and persistent, invasive, and ego-syntonic ideas of a sexual nature with self-referential characteristics: "I came to believe that people knew what was happening to me." His speech revolved around himself all the time, his incapacities and his fear of not being able to lead a normal life.

He spent his childhood in Angola, where he played outside the home frequently. From a very young age, he heard that sexuality was a natural thing, a part of normal development. He had his first intercourse at 13 and accompanied the older boys when they sought prostitutes. His dysfunctional sexual behavior became evident when he attended secondary school in Portugal. At the age of 16, he started to watch pornography in cyber cafés with a friend. His internet sex consumption progressively increased until he became obsessed with it. He classifies his behavior as "insatiable sex pursuit." Mr. S lost interest in softcore pornography early and moved to other forms, spending an average of 4 or more hours every day procuring and watching pornographic movies.

After he married, his behavior did not change, and this caused many marital conflicts. His wife became angry and accused him of carelessness in parental responsibilities. The situation worsened in such a way that his wife left him after filing a police complaint of domestic violence. Mr. S returned to the home of his elderly parents, who also did not accept that kind of behavior. Sometimes, even at work, he viewed pornographic movies and then masturbated in the bathroom; he often felt the need to have sex after leaving the office. Once he began, he would watch pornography for 4–5 hours continuously and occasionally throughout the night. He had developed features suggestive of mild depression, such as sadness, concentration difficulties, tiredness, feeling of unworthiness, decreased self-esteem, insomnia, and decreased appetite.

Past Sexual History

Before marrying, Mr. S sought prostitutes very often and never used a condom because it made him more sexually aroused. After the breakup of his marriage, he went 2 years without seeking intimacy with women. In recent months, he had started a relationship with a new girlfriend. One month before coming for consultation, he had made his first sexual advances with this girlfriend; however, he had not been able to perform due to erectile dysfunction. He kept comparing his girlfriend with females in pornographic videos, and he felt that she was not as sensual and attractive as the professional sex workers in them.

Treatment

Mr. S was started on fluoxetine 20 mg, titrated to 60 mg, as well as paliperidone, 3 mg/day. The latter was withdrawn after 60 days once his ideas of self-reference remitted. With sex education, his undue concerns about semen loss decreased significantly. He began cognitive-behavioral therapy and showed significant improvement after about 8 months of combined pharmacotherapy and psychotherapy. He felt much better on follow-up, and his compulsion to watch pornography had decreased significantly. Sometimes he could not resist the temptation and tried to view some images of pornographic content, but he never spent more than 30 minutes in this activity. His medication was gradually tapered, and both psychotherapy and pharmacotherapy were stopped after 24 months of treatment. He got married and had been doing well for more than a year. He was free from any sexual or mental health symptoms and receiving no treatment, coming in only for follow-up visits every 4 months.

Discussion

The conditioning role of culture in matters of sexual interest is best understood against the backdrop of the prohibitions in place in the relevant societies. Even in the absence of written laws, cultural taboos have a considerable impact on sexuality. Cultural mores and observances let us believe what may or may not be desired, what even if desired may or may not be pursued, and how our desires may or may not be expressed. Beliefs related to sexuality and the enactment of gender roles are deeply rooted in people's culture and history and in their relationships with others. For African men and their descendants, this sociosexual history includes a complex convergence of race, gender, sexual orientation, and socioeconomic status (Collins 2005). A stereotypical prejudice is that sexual activity among people from Africa is free, with no moral or religious value. Caldwell et al. (1989) claimed moreover that no religious moral value is attached to the sexual activity and that Christianity has not succeeded in changing this mindset. They find in this attitude the reason for the failure of fertility control programs in sub-Saharan Africa and argue that efforts to control HIV/AIDS will similarly fail unless the fear it generates forces Africans to adopt the Eurasian model, with its religious and moral values. However, as pointed out in many studies, sexual morality within the African context, as in other regions of the world, is also gender skewed (Oloruntoba-Oju 2007). The nontherapeutic alteration of children's genitals (female genital mutilation and male circumcision) is an example that reveals the extent to which dominant conceptions may be imbued with cultural values.

In the case of men, there is a continuity of the "male virile" discourse that "discards," "objectifies," and in turn constructs masculinity, sexuality, sexual identity, and the relationship with other sexualities. This type of representation leads men and women on the path to distancing themselves from affectionate and close people within the framework of their same sex and toward developing sexual relationships, becoming couples, and beginning a family (Nogueira 2008; Simon-Hohm 1986).

It is therefore not surprising that, in this case, adapting to the European way of life was not too distressing and disturbing. In Africa, Mr. S had a group of peers with whom he used to play in the street. Soon sexual experiences integrated into his normal development process (it is acceptable to admit an influence as cultural facilitator), although at home his parents' restrictive and negative view of sexual experiences was perpetuated by their religious beliefs. Objectively, moving to Europe for family reasons did not cause a noticeable discontinuity in his normal functioning; his academic performance remained adequate, and he enrolled at the university quickly.

The experience of living in Europe, among other things, facilitated Mr. S's access to new technologies and the internet. What stands out in this clinical case is the strong interdependence between access to the internet, the systematic consumption of pornography, and the consolidation of a pattern of behavior that was marked by sexual compulsivity. The internet may have triggered his latent compulsive behavior to become manifest.

Since childhood, Mr. S had always felt good about his body, and for him, the perception of an exacerbated libido was a natural and confirmatory aspect of his masculine identity. In many parts of Africa, virginity and widowhood customs continue to place a severe restriction on the actualization of female sexual desire, whereas men are not subject to such restrictions. This belief about African men that is rooted in the subconscious of people is reinforced by the images transmitted by the media of the exuberance of body worship, sensuality, and hedonism. The relatively high level of bodily exposure shown in the mass media, general dress codes, and substantial levels of public expression of affection reinforce such an image.

CONCLUSION

We agree with Silvia Ubillos et al. (2000) when they state that: "a culturalist explanation of sexuality will stress the importance of norms, values and principles in life, such as hedonism and personal autonomy in individualistic societies, and group loyalty and emotional dependence in collectivistic cultures" (p. 71). Clinical experience makes us understand that CSB is not caused by religious and other cultural factors, but these can play important roles. Cultural and religious determinants contribute but also enrich the complexity of these clinical cases.

REFERENCES

Alonso-Fernández F: La misoginia de don Juan Tenorio. Jano 63:36–41, 2002

Battiste M, Youngblood J: Protecting Indigenous Knowledge and Heritage: A Global Challenge. Vancouver, BC, Canada, UBC Press, 2000

Behere PB, Natraj GS: Dhat syndrome: the phenomenology of a culture bound sex neurosis of the orient. Indian J Psychiatry 26(1):76–78, 1984

Bellomo L: Erotomanía: la expresión clínica del delirio de ser amado. Alcmeón 12(1):18–33, 2005

Berger AA: The Art of the Seductress: Techniques of the Great Seductresses From Biblical Times to the Postmodern Era. Bloomington, IN, iUniverse, 2002

Berrios GE, Kennedy N: Erotomania: a conceptual history. Hist Psychiatry 13(52):381–400, 2002

Bhatia MS, Malik SC: Dhat syndrome: a useful diagnostic entity in Indian culture. Br J Psychiatry 159(5):691–695, 1991

Bhugra D, Popelyuk D, McMullen I: Paraphilias across cultures: contexts and controversies. J Sex Res 47(2–3):242–256, 2010

Boucé PG: Aspectos da tolerância e intolerância sexual na Inglaterra do séc. XVIII. Jornal para Estudos do Século XVIII 3(3)173–191, 1980

Bullough VL: The physician and research into human sexual behavior in nineteenth-century Germany. Bull Hist Med 63(2):247–267, 1989

Caldwell JC, Caldwell P, Quiggin P: The social context of AIDS in sub-Saharan Africa. Popul Dev Rev 15(2):185–234, 1989

Collins PH: Black Sexual Politics: African Americans, Gender, and the New Racism. New York, Routledge, 2005

Delugach SP: Indigenous models of healing and sexuality: restoring sexual balance. Sexual Addiction and Compulsivity 6(2):137–150, 1999

Diethelm O: Medical Dissertations of Psychiatric Interest Before 1750. Basel, Switzerland, Karger, 1971

Douglas M: Purity and Danger: An Analysis of Concepts of Pollution and Taboo. New York, Routledge, 2003

Edwards JW: Part 4: semen anxiety in South Asian cultures: cultural and transcultural significance. Med Anthropol 7(3):51–67, 1983

Esquirol E, Gayo C, Desviat M, García-Alejo RH: Memorias Sobre la Locura y Sus Variedades. Madrid, Spain, Dorsa, 1991

Giddens A: The Transformation of Intimacy: Sexuality, Love and Eroticism in Modern Societies. Hoboken, NJ, Wiley, 2013

Hirschfeld M: Sexual Anomalies: The Origins, Nature and Treatment of Sexual Disorders. New York, Emerson Books, 1948

Kar SK, Sarkar S: Dhat syndrome: evolution of concept, current understanding, and need of an integrated approach. J Hum Reprod Sci 8(3):130–134, 2015

Karaga S, Davis DE, Choe E, Hook JN: Hypersexuality and religion/spirituality: a qualitative review. Sexual Addiction and Compulsivity 23(2–3):167–181, 2016

Kirmayer L, Simpson C, Cargo M: Healing traditions: culture, community and mental health promotion with Canadian aboriginal peoples. Australasian Psychiatry 11(suppl):S15–S23, 2003

Massie RK: Catherine the Great: Portrait of a Woman. New York, Random House, 2012

Morgan K: No. 1 nation in sexy web searches? Call it Pornistan. Fox News, July 13, 2010

Murray KM, Ciarrocchi JW, Murray-Swank NA: Spirituality, religiosity, shame and guilt as predictors of sexual attitudes and experiences. Journal of Psychology and Theology 35(3):222–234, 2007

Nakra BS, Wig NN, Varma VK: A study of male potency disorders. Indian J Psychiatry 19(3):13–18, 1977

Nicholas LJ: The association between religiosity, sexual fantasy, participation in sexual acts, sexual enjoyment, exposure, and reaction to sexual materials among black South Africans. J Sex Marital Ther 30(1):37–42, 2004

Nogueira O: Color de piel y clase social. VIBRANT 5(1):XVII–LIV, 2008

Oloruntoba-Oju T: Body images, beauty culture and language in the Nigeria, African context. Presented at the Understanding Human Sexuality Seminar 2007 Series by the Africa Regional Sexuality Resource Center, University of Ibadan, Nigeria, September 13, 2007

Oosterhuis H: Stepchildren of Nature: Krafft-Ebing, Psychiatry, and the Making of Sexual Identity. Chicago, IL, University of Chicago Press, 2000

Pratt D: The Don Juan myth. American Imago 17(3):321–335, 1960

Ramazanoglu C (ed): Up Against Foucault: Explorations of Some Tensions Between Foucault and Feminism. Abingdon, UK, Routledge, 1993

Ranjith G, Mohan R: Dhat syndrome: a functional somatic syndrome? Br J Psychiatry 185(1):77, 2004

Simon-Hohm H: La socialización de los niños africanos: contradicción entre las normas sociales modernas y las tradicionales. Educar 9:23–34, 1986

Singh G: Dhat syndrome revisited. Indian J Psychiatry 27(2):119–122, 1985

Sophia EC, Tavares H, Zilberman ML: Pathological love: is it a new psychiatric disorder? (in Portuguese). Braz J Psychiatry 29(1):55–62, 2007

Sumathipala A, Siribaddana SH, Bhugra D: Culture-bound syndromes: the story of dhat syndrome. Br J Psychiatry 184(3):200–209, 2004

Trollope-Kumar K: Speaking through the body: leukorrhea as a bodily idiom of communication in Garhwal, India. Doctoral dissertation, McMaster University, 2001

Ubillos S, Paez D, González JL: Culture and sexual behavior. Psicothema 12(suppl):70–82, 2000

von Krafft-Ebing R: Psychopathia Sexualis: With Especial Reference to the Antipathic Sexual Instinct: A Medico-Forensic Study. New York, Arcade Publishing, 1998

Ware NC, Weiss MG: Neurasthenia and the social construction of psychiatric knowledge. Transcultural Psychiatric Research Review 31(2):101–124, 1994

Wilson K: Therapeutic landscapes and First Nations peoples: an exploration of culture, health and place. Health Place 9(2):83–93, 2003

Index

Page numbers printed in **boldface** type refer to tables and figures.